The Indispensable
Health Care Manager

The Indispensable Health Care Manager

Success Strategies
for a Changing Environment

Wendy Leebov
Gail Scott

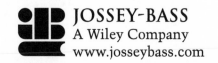

JOSSEY-BASS
A Wiley Company
www.josseybass.com

Published by

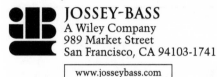

JOSSEY-BASS
A Wiley Company
989 Market Street
San Francisco, CA 94103-1741

www.josseybass.com

Jossey-Bass books and products are available through most bookstores. To contact Jossey-Bass directly, call (888) 378-2537, fax to (800) 605-2665, or visit our website at www.josseybass.com.

Substantial discounts on bulk quantities of Jossey-Bass books are available to corporations, professional associations, and other organizations. For details and discount information, contact the special sales department at Jossey-Bass.

We at Jossey-Bass strive to use the most environmentally sensitive paper stocks available to us. Our publications are printed on acid-free recycled stock whenever possible, and our paper always meets or exceeds minimum GPO and EPA requirements.

Credits are on page 269.

Library of Congress Cataloging-in-Publication Data
Leebov, Wendy.
    The indispensable health care manager : success strategies for
a changing environment / Wendy Leebov, Gail Scott.
        p. ; cm—(The Jossey-Bass health series)
Rev. ed. of: Health care managers in transition / Wendy Leebov,
Gail Scott. 1990.
Includes bibliographical references and index.
    ISBN 0-7879-6101-9 (alk. paper)
1. Health services administration
    [DNLM: 1. Administrative Personnel—United States. 2. Health
Services Administration—United States. 3. Organizational
Innovation—United States. W 84 AA1 L41i 2002] I. Scott, Gail,
1946– II. Leebov, Wendy. Health care managers in transition. III.
Title. IV. Series.
    RA971 . L37 2002
    362.1'068—dc21
    2001007677

first edition
HC Printing
10 9 8 7 6 5 4 3 2

Contents

Preface

Health care managers have needed versatile skills and fulfilled diverse roles for many years. The multiple functions managers have served, combined with the changing environment, make it hard to pinpoint how requirements of managers have evolved. We find ourselves in an increasingly turbulent and competitive environment, with greater diversity and generational differences among employees and customers creating new challenges. On top of that, beliefs about leadership are changing, as new trends define "the effective manager."

What have we required of health care managers over the years? And what has happened to these requirements? Managers feel swamped and besieged. Are they juggling more roles at once? Are they playing new and different roles? Or are there too few of them to do the demanding work that competes for their attention?

For years, we have been fascinated with the role of health care managers, because we think this role is pivotal to the health and success of health care organizations.

As far back as 1988, we set out to sight and map the far-reaching changes in this important role. At the time, through our work with the Einstein Consulting Group, we helped more than four hundred health care organizations develop and implement far-reaching service and quality improvement strategies in order to gain distinction by impressive service quality and a sustained culture of continuous improvement. While many organizations went all out to effect valuable improvements, the *long-term* effectiveness of these organizational change strategies seemed to depend substantially on the effectiveness of middle managers.

Time and time again, hopes were dashed and ambitious efforts thwarted at the point where middle managers needed to carry the ball. While many strategies blossomed in the capable hands of effective middle managers, others seemed to weaken or fizzle. Where results were disappointing, managers resisted doing what needed to be done, due to some combination of fuzzy expectations, lack of skill, disinterest, burnout, confusion, cynicism. In any case, we realized that if our clients (and therefore we ourselves) were going to be successful, we needed to mobilize managers to enter the domain of management roles and management performance.

In focus groups, site visits, interviews, and fieldwork, we listened and learned, ultimately drawing these conclusions. Until the mid-1980s, there was very little emphasis on leadership development in health care. Leaders were promoted from within, and because they were technically good at their jobs, executives assumed that they could run their departments and get their people to do what needed to be done. For a while this appeared to be true. But the environment became volatile and dynamic, bringing about changes in reimbursement, competition for customers, explosion in technology, specialization, and early signs of managed care, mergers, acquisitions, and system development. Add to this a growing tension between customers and providers, downsizing, periods of staffing shortages between one layoff and the next, increasing government regulation, litigation, unionization, and political winds blowing. An industry in chaos.

Health care leaders everywhere were in shock. Executives who saw change coming realized that they couldn't go it alone and worked hard to help their leadership teams develop the skills and resources to meet emerging challenges. Some succeeded, while others experienced a series of "programs of the month," achieving mediocre results at best.

While we agreed that managers desperately needed to become more flexible and versatile by expanding their skills, we realized that to focus on skills put the cart before the horse. Having worked closely with many managers, we posited that they no longer knew what was expected of them—that they were floundering as they brought old solutions to new problems. We decided to work on redefining what health care leaders needed to be—to develop a clear vision of their roles, with clearly defined behavioral expectations. Managers deserved this clarity and yearned for it.

The result was our book *Health Care Managers in Transition: Shifting Roles and Changing Organizations,* published by Jossey-Bass in July 1990. In that book, we described ten role shifts that managers needed to make in order to be successful, and we attempted to provide leaders with practical tools and techniques they could use to embrace their new role and the requisite behaviors. The book was and still is a best-seller for Jossey-Bass.

In the mid-nineties, our careers took different paths. Wendy left her job as president of the Einstein Consulting Group and became associate vice president, human resources, responsible for organization and staff development for Albert Einstein Healthcare Network. There, she worked with change processes in depth as a member of the senior administrative team. Then, in 1998, Wendy became vice president, human resources, for the Einstein network, where she continues to lead and support organizational change initiatives and specifically leadership development.

Gail became president of the Einstein Consulting Group after Wendy resigned and then left to start her own consulting practice in 1994. She and her team of consultants have concentrated heavily on finding new, innovative ways to help leaders gain the skills and supports they need to improve service to customers and create healthy productive workplaces. In the twelve years since we worked together on *Health Care Managers in Transition,* we have both interacted with thousands of leaders and hundreds of health care systems.

With continuing fascination with and respect for the role of health care managers in the performance of health care systems, we have stayed in touch and witnessed the *continued* evolution of their dynamic role. The pace of change has accelerated. There seems to be no breathing room between one change and the next or between the initiatives health care organizations must engage in to respond to the changing environment. Managers' plates are spilling over with priorities, often competing priorities, and everything has to be done yesterday. On top of that, downsizings, hospital failures, mergers, acquisitions, consolidations, divestitures, and other restructuring efforts have left many organizations in disarray, demoralizing managers and causing them to become jaded, cynical, even frightened in their so-called leadership positions.

Nurse managers now have hundreds of people reporting to them. Directors of support services and corporate services, thanks to consolidation efforts, are running several departments typically at several locations. Clinical managers have greater accountability for revenue and quality than ever. All of these managers have been hit by the tornado of changes and are now expected to respond with calmness, poise, skill, creativity, and effectiveness. Having been primarily the *receivers*, not the *initiators* of change, these managers have to now embrace new roles in order to not only cope and manage their own health and well being, but also to lead and manage their teams in alignment with the organization's priorities.

The health care division of Jossey-Bass insightfully recognized the tumult in health care leader roles and approached us about considering a rewrite of *Health Care Managers in Transition.* Thrilled with the prospect, we reread our own book and realized that it is surprisingly current. However, changes in the last ten years have precipitated even greater changes in managers' roles that merit dedicated and thorough attention. While some of the role shifts we identified in our earlier book still hold true, in this new book, we update and expand on these role shifts.

We define each shift and describe its importance. We make it real by applying it to real-life situations. We explore the costs and benefits managers experience when they make the transition to the new role. Then, we provide tools. For each shift, the first tools help the manager look at their own beliefs, attitudes, and internal dialogue or "self-talk," all with an eye to altering their mindset so that it drives them to behave in accord with their new role. Today's leaders must be more than willing; they must be hungry, eager, and available in their approach to their jobs. As we explore this mindset, we address the question, "How does the manager need to see their role? What beliefs about their role will serve them best, spurring them to behave in sync with the role shifts we present? Then, we provide *new and refreshing* tools managers can use to try on, try out, and internalize these role shifts in their everyday work.

We include dozens of examples and case studies in this new book. These are not fiction; we collected these from our work with leaders everywhere.

Rydal, Pennsylvania   Wendy Leebov
Meadowbrook, Pennsylvania   Gail Scott
November 2001

Acknowledgments

We want to express our deepest gratitude to all of our colleagues, clients, and staff members who have contributed to this book by sharing their trials, tribulations, successes, and learning with us. We are inspired by your determination, your hard work, your dedication, your many enlightening stories and profound insights. We are both happy to have been a part of your growth and development, as you have certainly been a powerful force in ours.

We also want to thank our families and friends for their contribution to our learning, their blind faith and lifelong encouragement. We especially want to thank Tom Quinlan and Julie Hyland for their help and generosity during the writing process. Thanks also to Julie Scenna Fitzgibbons, Mary Ellen Barnett, Florence Leebov, Linda Goldston, Lynda Rothman, Laura Brown, Pat Mathews, Todd Linden, Sparkles, Max, and Sophie for their enthusiastic support.

—W. L. and G. S.

The Authors

Wendy Leebov is vice president, human resources, for Albert Einstein Healthcare Network in Philadelphia and also founder and former president of the Einstein Consulting Group. She has more than twenty years' experience helping health care organizations design and launch organizationwide initiatives that advance service excellence and patient satisfaction, team effectiveness, and leadership competence. The author of numerous books, she has facilitated planning processes and presented speeches, teleconferences, and skill-building workshops for a variety of health care, public, and community organizations, as well as professional and voluntary associations. She also consulted with the Japanese Association of Medical Corporations on a national initiative to improve service quality in health care. Wendy received her doctorate in human development from the Harvard Graduate School of Education in 1971.

Gail Scott is president of Gail Scott and Associates, an international training and organizational development practice dedicated to helping health care leaders build and sustain learning organizations. An educator and consultant for more than twenty years, she is one of the most sought after speakers on customer satisfaction and leadership development and has worked with hundreds of national and local health care associations. Before starting her own consulting practice, she spent nine years as director of consulting services and three years as president of the Einstein Consulting Group. In the past two decades, she and her associates have worked with more than five hundred health care organizations nationwide, primarily in the areas of service quality, leadership development, and organizational change. She is also on the faculty of the American College of Healthcare Executives and currently is teaching two popular courses as well as a new offering based on material from this book.

The authors have collaborated on four best-selling books: *Health Care Managers in Transition: Shifting Roles and Changing Organizations* (Jossey-Bass); *Achieving Impressive Customer Service: Seven Strategies for the Healthcare Manager; Service Quality Improvement: The Customer Satisfaction Strategy for Health Care;* and *Patient Satisfaction: The Practice Enhancement Guide for Physicians.*

The Indispensable
Health Care Manager

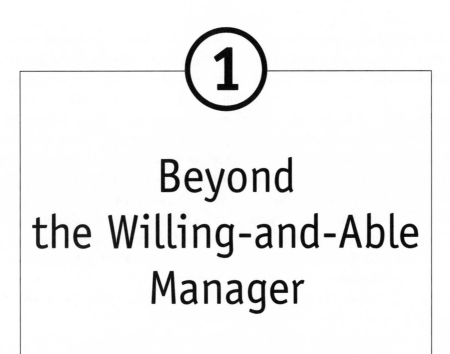

Beyond
the Willing-and-Able
Manager

The health care manager's job has never been easy. Like our colleagues in other industries, we want smooth-running, efficient systems. We want talented teams. We want innovation. And we want growth. But we want all of them in the *service* of our overarching mission: to help people get well, stay well, suffer as little as possible, and experience even the most trying and irreversible health challenges in the hands of people who offer dignity, comfort, compassion, and care. Like our colleagues in other industries, we want a strong bottom line. But in health care, a strong bottom line is a means to an end, rarely the end itself.

With this humanitarian mission front and center, health care management has attracted special people who have extraordinary commitment and dedication.

But these days, the job of health care manager demands superhero capabilities. The job requires commitment to mission for sure, but also visionary leadership, analytical skills, systems thinking, courage, persistence, creativity, agility, and the ability to mobilize and lead people. The job necessitates all this in an atmosphere of change and challenge that frequently feels overwhelming: changing rules, new entrants into the industry, hot competition that moves rapidly and strategically, plates spilling over with priorities, stress, competition with other employers for workers, financial constraints, changing rules and regs, systems coming together and falling apart, technology breakthroughs, media scrutiny, shifting demographics, accountability for quality and outcomes, requirements about patients' rights and privacy, and growing consumer savvy and vigilance.

A tall order? More like a skyscraper! Today's health care manager needs to be a versatile, flexible, multitalented leader.

Exhibit 1.1. Beyond Willing and Able.

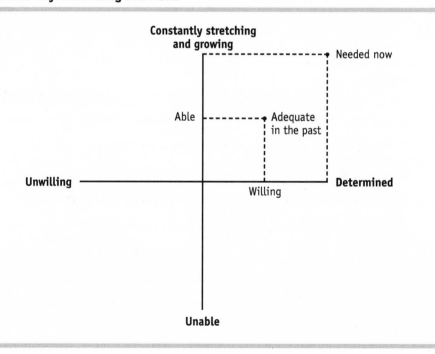

Nothing Short of a Squeeze

It used to be that health care managers needed to be willing and able. This was in contrast to being unwilling (resistant or cynical) and unable (lacking the needed competencies and skills). Now, even being willing and able isn't enough (Exhibit 1.1). More than willing, today's health care manager needs to be determined. More than able, today's health care manager needs to be constantly stretching and grow-ing—developing new capabilities all the time.

The pressures of today and the future combined with these ambitious demands on the role are provoking many a health care manager to take inventory. We are taking stock of ourselves. When we look within, some of us find feelings of excite-ment and challenge that we attribute to the stimulation of the complex, rapidly changing industry, to new opportunities—to learn, experiment, contribute. For others of us, these pressures trigger feelings of anxiety, inadequacy, fear, and fatigue.

In a management meeting recently, we asked managers to share metaphors that expressed how their job has been feeling lately. The resulting metaphors were won-derful—and telling.

- "In my job, I feel like *wilted lettuce thrown into ice water.* I was going along, perky and crisp. As time passed, I aged, of course—wilted, really. I got stale in my job, and all I wanted to do was get by and have a life outside of work. Then, the changes started happening in health care and in my hospital. That's when the wilted lettuce hit the ice water . . . and I perked up again from the shock of it."
- "In my job, I feel like my *bookshelf* at home. Like my bookshelf, I am *braced* to carry the weight. I have supports that prop me up under the weight of really heavy responsibilities. Some of these responsibilities, like my books, are old and dusty. Others are appealing and exciting. But there are a zillion of them, and I forget about most of them, instead paying attention to the ones that stand out."
- "In my job, I'm a *juggler,* but not an experienced one. I always have lots of balls in the air, and I always have lots of balls dropping. The problem is, I never get a break that allows me to catch the balls I dropped, because there are always more balls in the air."
- "I feel like a *rubber band*—one that breaks from constant stretching."
- "I feel like an *antique.* Enough said."
- "I feel like a *sponge.* I am absorbing so much and learning all the time."

- "I feel like a *truck in quicksand.* I wasn't paying attention and I swerved into the quicksand of this industry. Now, no matter how fast I gun my engine, I get in deeper—and I'm afraid of being swallowed up."
- "I feel like a *flagpole.* I really stand tall for some good values, but I'm planted in concrete. I like the way things were, and I hate the pressure to do things differently."
- "I feel like a *fire hydrant*—complete with dog."

Then there's *punching bag, blowup toy, caged animal, trash compactor, light bulb, tree.* . . .

The pressures are continuous. The demands on this role are diverse. The opportunities to stretch and learn are staggering. It requires not only talent but also internal strength and fortitude to feel good about our jobs—and adequate, let alone successful.

Ten Role Shifts That Make Us More Effective

To succeed in today's and tomorrow's health care environment, we need to stretch and grow in directions that necessitate changes in how we think and act.

Starting with how we think, the fact is that how we think drives our actions, priorities, decisions, and behavior. Our beliefs are the lens through which we view our work world. What we see and do as a result of looking at our work world through this lens has a giant impact on our effectiveness and value to the organization.

Here's an example. In the past, many of us believed that good employees are easy to find. With that belief or mind-set, a manager may very likely say no when asked to allow an employee some flexibility in his or her schedule—flexibility that is inconvenient for the manager to accommodate.

Today, this belief is proving problematic. Managers who think good employees are easy to find and therefore refuse to consider flexible scheduling are having problems retaining their best people. They are faced with crises and morale problems created by short staffing, and they use a lot of energy wracking their brains to find ways to recruit enough qualified people to fill key positions.

Here's another example. Some managers in the past thought they should move forward with a change, improvement, or new service only after they dotted every *i* and crossed every *t*. This led to some long, drawn-out decision-making processes and an eternity between an idea and its implementation. Today, speed is critical. In the face of an opportunity, it is impossible to dot every *i* and cross every *t* and still make a timely decision. If you apply slow, methodical, analytical decision-making processes to every opportunity, you miss many of them, because the competition moves faster and seizes the opportunity before you do.

Even if you have impressive skills and competencies, it's your mind-set that drives and motivates your behavioral choices. By changing your mind-set, you can change many behavior patterns at once, rather than one at a time. That makes it optimally efficient, in terms of your time and energy, to scrutinize your mind-set and then ask yourself if yours leads to the behavior and priorities you want. It is, after all, these behaviors and priorities that make the difference in your effectiveness.

To add value optimally to your organization—from the perspective of customers, staff, and leaders alike—ten role shifts are critical. These shifts (Exhibit 1.2) move us from ways of thinking and acting that were common, workable, and sufficient in the past to ways of thinking and acting that we must cultivate to be effective in today's environment and the future.

Exhibit 1.2. The Ten Role Shifts.

From	To
1. Provider orientation	Customer obsession
2. Silo thinking	Organizational perspective
3. Directing	Coaching
4. Status quo	Courage, risk, and change
5. Busyness	Results
6. Telling	Facilitating dialogue
7. Protecting turf	Building relationships
8. Function manager	Business leader
9. Employee as expendable	Employee as precious
10. Pressure and overwork	Balance and perspective

Shift One: From Provider Orientation to Customer Obsession

In the days when our health care organizations got paid for whatever services and time we decided to devote to patients, the patient did not exercise economic power over us. Most of us thought of ourselves as expert providers who could decide what would be best for our patients. We call this a "provider orientation." With competition, changes in reimbursement, and consumer awareness intensifying over the past years and decades, acting from the mind-set that "we know what's best for you" has lost its effectiveness. Patients now think of themselves as customers who can choose their provider and who have the right to demand involvement in decisions about quality, service, and value from that provider. If they don't get these things, they have the power to shift their business to the provider down the street.

With these changes, we in health care need to shift from a provider orientation to a customer orientation. Even that isn't enough. Because patients are vulnerable and fearful, we have a special responsibility to take exceptional care of them and do all we can to enhance their experience while they are in our hands. These days, and in the future, an obsession with customer satisfaction must replace a customer orientation. As health care managers, we have to embrace this obsession in our minds and act from it in how we manage our areas of responsibility and how we focus and coach our teams.

Shift Two: From Silo Thinking to Organizational Perspective

It used to be relatively uncomplicated: people worked in a department in a hospital. Now, it's more likely that people work in a subsidiary or department of a hospital that's one of several in a network that may be part of a system with other networks. Huh? It's no surprise that people wonder to themselves *Where do I fit?* It doesn't work anymore to be focused only on your immediate world, your department or your facility. Picture a silo on a farm: the tall building with high walls that protect what's within from the elements. A department or facility that has a silo mentality these days runs the risk of tunnel vision, which leads to action and decisions that run against the grain of the organization's best interest. The health care manager today must "think organization" and look and reach beyond the immediate domain to relate to the other parts of the complex whole in order to add maximum value to the organization.

Shift Three: From Directing to Coaching

Maybe it's a style or generational thing. It used to be that directing was the prevalent management style in organizations; they were strong on hierarchy and authority lines were solid, with some people being the bosses and some people being the subordinates. Not only has our language changed but also new generations have entered our workforce that are less tolerant of a management style characterized by authority and control. Increasingly, they expect respect for the expertise and talent they bring. They want room to participate meaningfully, and they want to grow and learn on the job.

Directing used to work, but now it works well only in situations that require an immediate decision. Directing may work in certain situations, but coaching on the manager's part tends to bring about not only better results and greater responsibility on the part of the employee but also a more satisfied, gratified employee.

Shift Four: From Status Quo to Courage, Risk, and Change

Before our society sped up to today's feverish pitch, health care organizations survived year after year without having to install or undergo much change. We could do things as we always had and create the results we always did and enjoy the rewards we always enjoyed. But no more. With computers, technological breakthroughs, mergers, restructuring, buyouts, partnering, competition, system formation, the Internet, and other now-commonplace forces of change, the status quo equates with stagnation. The status quo–oriented organization can expect to fall, while the organization with managers who are courageous, risk-taking, and changeworthy move ahead.

Shift Five: From Busyness to Results

In the era when the health care organization was relatively free of pressure to implement one change after another, a manager experienced less pressure to produce results. Staying busy and managing one's responsibilities in a reliable and competent way sufficed. Not today; we are pressed to demonstrate our value by achieving results—lots of them, and quickly. We have lost the luxury of time. If we do not move quickly enough and produce results, our competitors leave us in the dust.

Shift Six: From Telling to Facilitating Dialogue

"Here's how it's going to be."

"Our board has completed our plan, and I'm here to tell you about it."

"I've developed some new rules for our work team, and here they are."

In the past, statements like these were common, reflecting the popular management style of the era: telling. Today, telling isn't as effective. For one thing, no boomer, generation Xer, or nexter appreciates it as an exclusive approach. Research about all three of these generations (which we mention again in Chapter Seven) indicates that their members want meaningful participation in decisions. They want influence; they want to be heard. They know they have valuable thoughts and ideas, and they want their managers to respect them by inviting their involvement.

On top of this, the complexity and speed of our health care environment make it wise for a health care manager to tap every possible ounce of talent and creativity available. A telling management style doesn't welcome, or even allow, the best ideas, perspective, and thinking of everyone on the team. In today's environment, the manager has to become a facilitator of dialogue. We need to have lots of ways to invite our staff, colleagues, customers, teachers, neighbors, vendors, and so on to engage with us about the challenges we face, the dynamics we must understand, the goals we must embrace, and the decisions we need to make. Becoming a dialogue facilitator is a real stretch for lots of us, but one that reaps amazing benefits for the sake of the manager, employee retention, and value added to the organization's mission.

Shift Seven: From Protecting Turf to Building Relationships

"Circle the wagons and the enemy can't get in." That's an exaggerated way to describe the turf protection that typified the health care manager in the past. Many managers guarded their people and their functions zealously, keeping others out to have maximum control and also to prevent others from meddling, criticizing, or second-guessing. This really didn't create much of a problem. Most everyone behaved this way. We learned turf protection from our own managers, and we carried on the tradition. But today, we need cooperation, partnerships, and support beyond our immediate domain. We cannot be effective by circling the wagons. We have to actively and proactively form strong relationships with our own staff; with people in other departments and services; and with customers, community members, vendors, and many others beyond our organization. If we don't form such relationships, we operate in a relative vacuum and cannot be effective in our decisions or responsive in our service.

Shift Eight: From Function Manager to Business Leader

Running a hospital department in the days when change was not the norm was largely a custodial function. Departmental practices had been in place and working. The effective manager tended the store and made sure the department continued to fulfill its functions and contribute to the overall workings of the organization. But in our change-frenzied world, running a department and keeping things going smoothly is only a minor, albeit important, aspect of the job. Whether a department is a cost center or a revenue center, today's health care manager needs to think and act like a business owner or entrepreneur, with responsibility for innovation and improvement, cost control, and revenue enhancement. He or she is responsible for every facet of the business and maximizing its value to the organization at large. This requires entirely different skills from those of the functional manager.

Shift Nine: From Employee-as-Expendable to Employee-as-Precious

A manager cannot get along without talented, committed staff. In the heyday of plenty, the health care manager could hire workers easily and fill positions quickly with talented people. Ah, for the good old days. Today, there is a global talent shortage, as well as specific and severe shortages of qualified health care workers in an increasing variety of fields: nursing, pharmacy, radiology, psychiatry, speech therapy, health care accounting, and many more.

The fact is, no longer can you expect to fill vacant positions easily. No more can you assume access to a pool of talented staff at affordable rates. The consequence is that it pays to consider every employee you have as a precious gem; you must do everything possible to polish that precious gem so it stays in your organization and continues to enable you to serve your patients. The manager who treats staff as expendable loses them and ends up bereft of the talent needed to provide critical services.

Shift Ten: From Pressure and Overwork to Balance and Perspective

Running ragged. Rushing around like a chicken with your head cut off. Busy, busy, staying long hours, giving your work your all. Working in an atmosphere of pressure, overload, and overwork drains your batteries. In today's (and tomorrow's) environment, the challenges are so great that every one of us must maintain balance and perspective or else burn out. When we burn out, we lose our stamina and stick-to-itiveness; we reduce our work effectiveness and also pay a price in our lives (if we have a life outside of work). Survival in today's health care environment requires balance and perspective. As managers, we need to demonstrate this in our own lives for the sake of our health and performance—and also for our precious staff members, who themselves want and deserve to have balance in their own lives.

New Requirements in the Face of Change

Listing the ten shifts, with the old way in the left-hand column and the new way in the right-hand column, would be an easy way to portray things, but it may be misleading. Resist the temptation to think bad or wrong about the old patterns. They were typical, accepted, taught, and learned in past years; they worked. The managers who operated accordingly felt effective. Those of us in health care jobs experienced the old patterns from our own managers and learned them as we grew from young pups to seasoned managers. Our point is that these accepted, learned patterns have lost their resilience. Except in limited situations, they don't work so well in the emerging health care environment.

Hot competition, rising quality, safety, and outcome standards, worker shortages, HIPAA, consumer scrutiny, technology changes, resource constraints, and speed are the norm. No wonder some old ways don't work as well anymore. Effective managers of the past need to revolutionize their roles to meet the demands of a new world.

Listing these shifts in two columns may mislead you in another way. These patterns are not either-or. They are really on a continuum. Some people think and act the same way from situation to situation, but many more are flexible and capable of moving from one point to another along the continuum.

For instance, consider the continuum from telling to facilitating dialogue. In a crisis situation, you might be inclined to tell people what they are to do. On the other hand, in planning a project in which you want to engage your staff, you might be inclined to invite and foster dialogue and the investment in the plan that this would probably inspire. How you think and act related to these shifts may be situational. It might also depend on the degree of consciousness with which you choose how you want to think and act. Sometimes people think the "old" way under pressure: they act from their patterns. When they are more relaxed and have a chance to think through what they're about to do, they might think in a new way. The difference is conscious choice. Ideally, you revisit your habitual ways of thinking and responding, assess their consequences, and as needed work to build new habits. Eventually, your prevalent style or pattern, or modus operandi, shift to conform spontaneously, consistently, and painlessly to the new role demands.

The Question: Are You Where You Want to Be?

Do the quick self-appraisal in Exhibit 1.3 just to get an idea of your current mind-set profile.

Exhibit 1.3. Your Current Profile: Where Are You on Each Continuum?

Provider orientation	1	2	3	4	5	6	Customer obsession
Silo thinking	1	2	3	4	5	6	Organizational perspective
Directing	1	2	3	4	5	6	Coaching
Status quo	1	2	3	4	5	6	Courage, risk, and change
Busyness	1	2	3	4	5	6	Results
Telling	1	2	3	4	5	6	Facilitating dialogue
Protecting turf	1	2	3	4	5	6	Building relationships
Function manager	1	2	3	4	5	6	Business leader
Employee-as-expendable	1	2	3	4	5	6	Employee-as-precious
Pressure and overwork	1	2	3	4	5	6	Balance and perspective

On the basis of this quick self-appraisal, which two shifts do you consider to be your strengths?

1. _____

2. _____

Which two do you consider to be developmental opportunities for you?

1. _____

2. _____

Repositioning Yourself for the Future

If you have assessed your own position relative to the ten role shifts and find that you want to change, then you *can.* You have the power to alter how you think and act. But you may be thinking, *I can't do this. My work culture doesn't encourage the ways of thinking and acting Wendy and Gail are suggesting.*

That may be true. Some executive teams, bosses, and health care cultures do encourage managers to function in new ways and encourage them through word and deed to make the transition. If this describes your culture, wonderful! Consider yourself lucky. But others don't. Instead, managers who want to be significant contributors and set the pace for progress hit their heads against the wall, when executive rhetoric—but not executive support—is consistent with the intended changes.

Your ability to succeed in your role and to achieve great results by operating in the new way certainly does depend partly on the leadership, practices, incentives, and culture of your organization. But rest assured, we have seen maverick after maverick change to the new ways and show bosses and colleagues better results.

If you choose to change your ways of thinking to better align with the new role demands, you will find this book packed with strategies and tools to help you make the shifts. In the last chapter, we identify some organizational supports that help you make the transition if your leaders are so inclined. Hopefully, you'll make explicit how you want to think and act and lobby for their support.

It's Better to Wear Out Than Rust Out

Even if you do recognize the importance of embracing the new role demands, you might be apprehensive about your ability to make the needed changes or about having the energy required in the stretch to new ways of thinking and behaving. Include these points in any pep talk you might repeat to yourself often:

- If you keep renewing yourself and learning, you earn people's respect.

- You become more versatile, able to handle the mix (or mess) of situations you're likely to face.

- If you willingly change to the new ways, you do not deplete your energy by holding on to the old ways. You free up your energy to learn and grow and enhance your results.

- If you rise to the occasion and learn the new ways, you renew yourself in your work. Forget being frantic, bored, tired, or cynical. Your days will be filled with challenge, stimulation, refreshing energy, and accomplishments.

- The health care environment is nuts! If you expand your versatility and cultivate new ways of thinking and acting, you have a better chance of surviving the turbulence and making valued contributions.

- Rising to meet the new role demands means challenge, stretch, learning, renewal, and new possibilities and opportunities, if you do so with energy, optimism, and speed.

- It's better to wear out than rust out. Changing yourself can be stressful and anxiety-provoking, but it's better than the alternative.

Finally, a word about optimism. The health care industry is fraught with challenges and pressures. It doesn't require rocket science to detect strain, stress, and cynicism on the faces and in the hearts of many managers today. These conditions make the call to change a grueling proposition.

We think optimism is a decision—a choice. It isn't an inevitable consequence of external conditions. Looking at the same glass, one person might see it as half empty while a second might see it as half full. A third might see it as not only half full but with room for more.

To embrace and internalize even one of the role shifts we identify here, you must adopt the positive expectation that you can make needed changes in both your thinking and your actions. You have to believe that you can amass the support you require to make and sustain these changes.

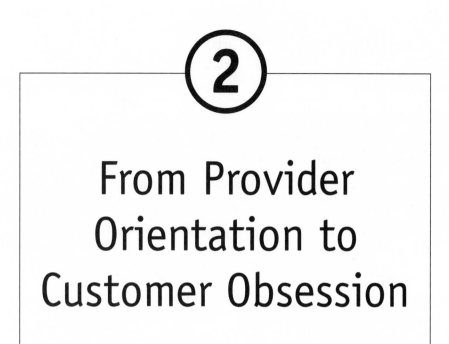

From Provider Orientation to Customer Obsession

Ⓢavvy consumers with a scrutinizing eye, severe resource constraints that compel us to focus attention on the bottom line, hot competition—all of these propel us toward adoption of a customer orientation, expressed in relentless determination to meet our customers' needs and impress them with our services. This takes more than a customer orientation. It takes an obsession with customer satisfaction.

A Revealing Look in the Mirror

True or False?	True	False
1. I have identified and made my staff aware of expectations our internal and external customers have of our services.	___	___
2. I have systems in place to measure customer satisfaction.	___	___
3. I routinely involve my staff in activities related to service improvement.	___	___
4. I have created specific guidelines and standards for the way that my team and I treat our customers.	___	___
5. I hold myself and others accountable to standards of excellence.	___	___
6. I don't think it is possible to meet the demands of today's unreasonable customer.	___	___
7. I believe that people either have it or they don't when it comes to dealing with customers.	___	___
8. When I bring new people onto my team, I am more concerned about their technical skills than their customer service skills.	___	___
9. Quite honestly, I am more concerned with the bottom line than I am with pleasing my customers.	___	___
10. I feel powerless to make a difference when it comes to satisfying customers.	___	___

If you answered true to the first five questions and false to the last five, you are clearly driven by a customer orientation. You see customer satisfaction as central to your role, and you structure many aspects of your job to pursue excellence in this arena. Some people might even say that you are obsessed with the need to satisfy customers. You establish service standards and consciously coach your staff to meet or exceed them. You have measures of customer satisfaction in place and hold yourself and your team accountable. You feel empowered to meet customer expectations. And you engage your staff in the process.

If this is true, we applaud you. Although many managers understand conceptually why they should care about customers, few have aligned their roles and activities with this focus. Why is that?

It's a New Day

Health care organizations have taken customer satisfaction and customer loyalty for granted. Until recently, people in health care avoided using the word *customer* in referring to patients, or any other customers (such as referral sources, physicians, community members, plan members, and the like). *Customer* has been and still is taboo in many organizations because of our provider orientation, which reveals itself in such beliefs as these:

- We are the experts.

- As health care providers knowledgeable about health care and people, we know what is good for the patient.

- As professionals who care about the patient, we do what is right for the patient even when the patient may not know what that is.

- We heal and save lives. Patients should be grateful for all that we do for them.

Do you hear some paternalism in a provider orientation? The health care field has been undergoing tumultuous change. We are all competing for patients, managed care contracts, and staff. Public perception has shifted. People no longer think of the health care organization and those who work in it as the good guys, with their best interests at heart. Consumers view us as focused only on the bottom line, denying care, making mistakes, and necessitating control and regulation. The new consumer is more demanding. Having been to Disney World and Nordstrom, where customers receive red-carpet treatment, people expect more from their health care providers. They are educated; they go online for information, shop for the best, and aggressively seek information from family and friends. They believe they deserve humane treatment and top-notch service and want value for their money. We're operating in a different world.

Some of us may be playing catch-up and have a long way to go. Because of a tradition of provider-oriented thinking, we may not have paid adequate attention to the patient as customer. Many of our systems and processes have not been designed with their comfort and expectations in mind. Many of us have not thought to research what our customers need and want, or to review the established expectations and standards that deliver it to them. We may not have adequately fostered a customer orientation and clear service expectations with our own staff. We may not have feedback systems in place that regularly reveal from our customers what they think of our services, or we may collect data but fail to scrutinize them and use customer feedback to drive service improvement.

Now, you might be thinking that what we've just said does not apply to your organization or system, because your group has been focusing time, resources, and energy on customer service and satisfaction. But we've seen many organizations, having established this as a priority, that are yet to emphasize that it is *up to you the manager.* Or even if your higher-ups have said the words, they may not have given you the opportunity or support to build the skills that turn a customer obsession into an impressive level of customer satisfaction. Executives might think global when they advance customer service as the strategic priority it deserves to be, but impressive service is a matter of design at the local level. *You* are the driver of impressive service. You make it happen in your team, and between your team and its multiple customers.

Take a Look

To move beyond rhetoric, let's see how managers with a provider orientation and those with a customer obsession approach everyday situations quite differently.

Tina

Tina is manager of a busy emergency department. She has been receiving complaints about long waits, the unattractive and unpleasant waiting area, the restrictive visitor's policy, rude and indifferent employees, and lack of teamwork with other departments. She knows that her team members have endured many changes—in leadership, and short-staffing resulting in demanding workloads, inconsistent service quality, and diminishing resources. Because of these circumstances, she feels powerless to make the changes she would like to make, and she knows that the plans to remodel the emergency department are several years down the road. As you can imagine, this is not helping staff and physician morale, and it is not making patients happy.

With her provider orientation, Tina thinks, *Why are people picking on us? We aren't the only ones with problems around here.* She might also fall into the trap of thinking that there are so many problems, so many issues to deal with, that nothing she does makes a difference. She offers excuses for staff, saying "They're too busy, volumes are impossibly high, the environment isn't supportive, it's someone else's fault." She does not have to deal with staff behavior, because she accepts their frustration as a reason the standards cannot be raised. In short, as a provider-oriented manager, Tina feels like a victim.

On the other hand, as a customer-obsessed manager, she does not regard doing nothing as an option. She recognizes that doing nothing means dropping behind competitors and failing to meet customers' heightening expectations. She develops a personal service mission and vision of excellence that she communicates clearly and often, to focus staff on customer needs and ever-higher standards of service. She helps staff understand that, although they are not to blame for many service problems, they can still bring about solutions and indeed have a responsibility to do so. She insists that even small improvements make a difference to customers. She observes how things are working, and she works hard to perceive service interactions from a customer's point of view to identify improvements. She creates and oversees implementation of a long-term plan to engage her staff in making service improvements, one step at a time.

Tom

Tom is in charge of several support departments. Managers and staff in other departments view him and his team as customer-unfriendly. Neither Tom nor his team have previously participated in the customer service strategy in his system. When asked to participate, Tom says, "My staff doesn't interact with patients, and neither do I. This isn't for us."

As a provider-oriented manager, Tom doesn't identify with the notion that we are each other's customers. He doesn't accept that, just as clinical services are judged by their customers, his departments have internal customers whose expectations they need to meet. He doesn't see it this way. He has not shared anything different with his team.

In today's environment, Tom is opting out as an important contributor to the organization's service mission. Even if he works in a system that has not engaged him in its customer service strategy, if he were a customer-obsessed manager he would take the initiative to get closer to his internal customers. He would talk to them about their needs, asking "How are we doing? What are we doing well? What do you need us to do better?" and use this input to redesign services, processes, and procedures with the customer in mind.

As a customer-obsessed manager, Tom knows that even if you aren't serving patients directly, you are serving people who do. He gets involved in planning service strategies in clinical areas beyond his own. He wants to help, knowing that the organization is only perceived as impressive when every department or division offers top-notch service.

Pearl

Pearl has several long-term subordinates who may be technically competent but are known as problem employees. They generate complaints from patients and families, and they cause problems for other employees. But they have ties in the community as well as strong relationships with several physicians.

As a provider-oriented manager, she doesn't feel comfortable about rocking the boat or equipped to do so. She doesn't confront employees because of their ties to important people or because she is afraid she might alienate or anger them.

If Pearl were a customer-obsessed manager, she would not be satisfied with a good-enough team. She would know that a few problem people keep the entire group from excelling at service. She would create clear standards of service excellence and hold everyone to the same standards. The interesting twist is that Pearl knows how to use peer pressure as a way to get through to people who have been holding the team and customers hostage. She also uses feedback and measurement to drive change and makes sure that everyone on her team gets meaningful feedback on their performance.

What Worries You?

Are you finding yourself saying "Yes, but . . ." at the thought of devoting energy to becoming more customer-obsessed? We've heard managers voice many understandable concerns about making this shift.

Are you concerned about asking your team to improve when they feel so stretched and worn out? You can't improve service on your own. You need your team to join you in this pursuit. That means you have to *sell* the importance of customers and service quality to your people. They need to know why the team needs to improve, what's in it for customers, and what's in it for them. This isn't an easy sell in today's environment. You need to address staff concerns in a way that keeps them engaged and overcomes any "no way, no how" resistance.

Are you concerned about the amount of time customer-driven pursuits take from you when you have so much on your plate? Once you open the discussion, you need to join, engage, and coach your team, and you have to follow through. Your team is involved in the improvement process, and they need your support. This takes time and commitment on your part.

Are you worried about other managers who might shun you if you raise the standards of service in the face of their inattention to service issues? Inevitably, there are people in most organizations who clearly don't want to pursue service improvement. These individuals may be threatened by you if you step up your attention to service quality and customer satisfaction. You may have to prepare to handle their active or passive resistance. You may need to help these individuals get on board by giving them direct feedback, whether they ask for it or not.

Is this just one more fish in the sea of priorities? You are already busy. You have other problems to attend to. The truth is, everyone is concerned with the financial realities and pressures facing health care. We are all worried about survival, and we get this message daily from our bosses. It's hard to focus on customers when we are consumed with making our budgets work, growing our business, filling vacancies with qualified people, keeping our staff happy, and the like.

Are you worried about keeping service improvement ongoing and getting lost in the process? You may not be comfortable with the process and the amount of time it takes to create change. If you are a person who wants to see quick results, ongoing attention to service problems, especially the tough ones, could drive you batty. Creating a culture of continuous improvement in your area takes time. It requires that you and your people do a lot of things at once. It isn't a linear process, and there is no roadmap or recipe. You and your group need to adopt an experimenter mind-set and be willing to do what it takes, learning and making course corrections along the way.

What Do You Stand to Gain?

It's not easy to remain calm about the benefits of shifting to a customer orientation. The fact is, the two of us authors have both been obsessed with the importance of customer satisfaction for years and have devoted considerable sweat to promote and advance it. We know that when managers and their teams embrace this obsession, they do a better job for patients and other customers. They are happier with each other and their work. It's an obsession that produces win-win benefits for all concerned.

Our obsession aside, consider what you stand to gain from joining us in our customer obsession.

- *Satisfied customers become loyal customers.* It is much easier to retain customers than to attract new ones. When you create a pattern of customer satisfaction, your customers not only choose your services but also tell others about them and become your most powerful and least costly marketing tool.

- *Happier customers are easier to serve.* It's quite simple. When people are satisfied with the service you provide, they are more cooperative and complain less. You have fewer angry customers. You have fewer frustrations to address and resolve. When these happy customers spread the word that your service is great, others come to you expecting great service. This sets up a positive rather than negative chain of events. Even if something goes wrong, if customers are disappointed, their problems are easier to solve because they already believe that you care.

- *Managers who care about customers attract talented staff.* When you and your people gain a reputation for excellence, you attract a higher-caliber employee. People really do want to work for a manager who cares about customers and wants to deliver great service to them. They know they'll feel proud of being part of the team.

- *You see results, and they give you relief.* In the process of designing service improvements and establishing unbeatable service standards, you create opportunities to address issues that have been a thorn in your side for years. You also propel yourself and others to confront individuals on your team who drag down the standards. It's like cleaning out a closet. It's work, but you like how it looks and feels as you see progress. Do you have some resisters hiding in your closet, people you have been avoiding and working around for years? By adopting a customer obsession, you are much more likely to deal with them; you end up feeling much better about your contribution to your organization and its mission.

- *You earn people's respect.* When you offer great service and engage your staff in the process, you gain the respect of those peers whom you respect, as well as that of your bosses—and most important, your staff. In the long run, they thank you for taking a stand and raising the standards. By taking the service bull by the horns, you do your part, and your supporters thank and appreciate you.

• *You learn, learn, learn.* In the process of applying your customer obsession to create effective processes, solutions, and happy customers, you learn a great deal about yourself and your team. All of you develop new skills, are more marketable and employable, and earn respect as the team to watch—the pacesetters, the team at the cutting edge.

What Can You Do? How Can You Do It?

We hope you are convinced that you have much to gain by developing a customer-driven approach; to support you, we offer three doable strategies.

First, we help you examine your thinking and compare and contrast it with the thinking of a customer-obsessed manager. Because change must begin with you, we also help you examine your commitment to excellence. If you don't decide to stretch your expectations of yourself and others, you won't be driven to do what a customer-obsessed manager does.

Second, because we are so close to our services that we lose sight of the details, and because customers come to us with certain expectations that are vital to their satisfaction, we share techniques you can use to get in close touch with your customers, so you can then use what you learn to celebrate successes and, in the face of problems, make course corrections.

Finally, because you can't satisfy customers alone, we include tools to help you make your customer obsession contagious, engaging your team in caring about customer satisfaction deeply and making improvement after improvement.

Although our book *Achieving Impressive Customer Service* has a much more comprehensive toolkit, the three strategic tools we share here (Exhibit 2.1) get you moving. They are practical and easy to implement, and they get results.

Exhibit 2.1. Your Customer Obsession Toolkit.

Strategy one: Think your way into a customer obsession.

Strategy two: Get close to your customers.

Strategy three: Engage your team.

Strategy One: Think Your Way into a Customer Obsession

Do you often have such thoughts as *I can't do this*, *This is not my job*, or *It won't matter anyway*? We shared some of the behaviors of the customer-obsessed manager in the true-false quiz and case situations, but what *thinking* drives those behaviors? In our work with managers, we've found time after time that those who run customer-driven teams and services hold a set of beliefs that move them to do customer-oriented things, that shape the way they interact with their customers and their teams.

First, the customer-obsessed leader regards customer satisfaction as critical to success. These leaders understand that in today's competitive environment they can't afford to disappoint customers. For them, being pretty good is not good enough.

These managers also accept responsibility for influencing the beliefs of the team members. They know that if they don't reserve and protect time for service improvement, it won't happen. It isn't up to the Human Resources Department or the Training Department. It is up to them.

The customer-obsessed leader also believes that consistent service that meets customer needs is possible; the leader can make a difference with staff through unrelenting focus on customers.

Do you think like a customer-obsessed leader? Or do you hold beliefs and think thoughts that stop you from dedicating your skills and energy to meeting customer needs?

If you aren't 100 percent convinced that you will benefit from a customer obsession, you are not able to display and communicate passion and commitment; nor are you able to sell this commitment to your team. Our first exercise helps you realize the price you may be paying if you're holding on to a provider orientation. Specifically, you'll see how much time and energy you spend during the day because service is *not* wonderful and your customers are not happy.

⚒ Tool: How Do You Spend Your Time? (Tool from Scott, 1999)

Purpose. This tool helps you analyze how you spend your time and gain appreciation for the amount of time that you spend reacting to customer problems and complaints.

Method. On a piece of paper, create two columns. Think about your past week.

In the first column, list all the times that you and your people dealt with unhappy customers. Think of your internal as well as external customers. Briefly describe the issue or incident.

In the second column, estimate the time you and others spent addressing the problem or complaint. (See example below.)

Look over your list. Ask yourself, *How would my week have been different if we had prevented these problems in the first place?*

An Example

Incident	Time
Mrs. Jones lost her teeth.	2 hours
Dr. Smith was upset because he wasn't notified of a change in the schedule.	30 minutes
Sue was upset with Rachael for not letting her know that she intended to leave early.	30 minutes
Mr. Smith forgot to reschedule his appointment but came in anyway.	20 minutes

After you take a crack at this, consider the time and energy spent in one week on customer problems and complaints. We've found in discussions with managers that many assume that a certain level of complaints is par for the course, expected, normal, unavoidable. Yet their analysis of their time (and perhaps yours) shows the daily wear and tear on them and their team of having to react to problems left unsolved, service snags that frustrate customers, and in-your-face complaints.

Many of these problems could and should be avoided. Customers are not getting what they need in the first place. The pressure to deal with emerging complaints and issues creates the stresses that are at the heart of burnout and low morale. Most of us want to do a good job, and when a problem rears its ugly head—especially if we know the problem is unnecessary—we get discouraged and depressed. We know that we aren't spending our time on the things that could make a positive difference to customers and staff.

This next tool takes your thinking one step further. It asks you to think about groups or stakeholders in your organization and what each one has to gain by focusing more on customers. Think about these questions by yourself first. Later, we describe how you can share the same questions with your staff. It is a wonderful way to create a rationale for change. Remember, the customer-obsessed leader believes the obsession for customer satisfaction produces benefits for everyone except competitors.

 ### Tool: Who Benefits? (Leebov, Scott, and Olson, 1998)

Purpose. This tool helps you think about the benefits for various stakeholders in focusing your mind and actions on identifying, meeting, and exceeding customer needs.

Method. Think about your customer groups and how each group would benefit by receiving top-notch, award-winning service.

Consider benefits for:

- You, the manager
- Your entire team
- Your patients and internal customers
- Physicians
- The community
- The organization

Of the benefits listed, identify those you feel most strongly about, and tell why.

Now, imagine you're about to get on a soapbox and give a one-minute speech about why it is critical to operate from a customer obsession. Cite the benefits that you find compelling.

To reinforce thinking as a customer-obsessed manager, keep a firm grip on these benefits; they strengthen your driving beliefs and your resolve to improve your customer obsession and keep customer needs at the forefront.

Having aligned your thoughts with a customer obsession, what can you actually do to internalize this obsession into your approach to the job?

Strategy Two: Get Close to Your Customers

Believing in a customer obsession is important, but the belief has to be detectable from your priorities, your activities, and the yardsticks to evaluate your effectiveness. We think a critical first step is, to the extent possible, to adopt your customer's perspective. You are, after all, an experienced customer who has sometimes been satisfied and sometimes disappointed, and who knows the difference. This next tool asks you to delve into your own experience as a customer, to identify what matters most to you.

You have been on the receiving end of the kind of wonderful service that results when a service team or organization holds customer satisfaction sacred. Perhaps you haven't considered the thought and design work that makes this wonderful service happen. By consciously considering your experience as an impressed customer and imagining the work behind the scenes, you can gain ideas about possibilities for improvement in your area.

⚒ Tool: Think of a Place (Leebov, Scott, and Olson, 1998)

Purpose. This tool applies your own experience and insights as an impressed customer to setting priorities for service improvement for your customers.

Method. Close your eyes and think about a place where you have been on the receiving end of impressive service—a place where you have been, to say the least, a satisfied customer. Just let your mind wander as you revisit your experience in a place that values its customers.
Take a few minutes to reflect on the things that impress you. Think about the environment, the systems, and the people. What exactly do people say and do to let you know that you are important?

Jot down on a piece of paper:

- What impressed you, and why
- What impressed you about the people and how you were treated?
- What is it about the environment, policies, or systems that impressed you?
- On the basis of what you appreciated in this experience, what would you like to do better or differently for your customers?

Did you have an easy time pinpointing the things you value as a customer? Think about this in the next few weeks. Be an astute observer whenever you are in a public place. In a store or restaurant, listen to what people say, and watch what they do when they are (or are not) taking care of you.

A caution: really looking at service quality and behavior toward customers in your own experience as a customer tends to become a habit. As you become more attuned and attentive, you may find yourself unable to enjoy the neighborhood restaurant or shopping experience. But know that you will learn a great deal from becoming conscious of and thoughtful about the service you're receiving and the management thinking and behavior that led to it. We promise that you will never take service for granted again, and you will strengthen your own customer obsession as a result.

Whoa, just a minute! Even though tuning in to your own experience as a customer is highly educational, we're cautioning you about the danger of generalizing about *your* customers from your own experience. *I know what my customers experience; I don't need to ask* is a thought that reflects a provider orientation more than customer obsession.

Your next step is to make sure you understand what *your* customers want and need from you, and how they feel as they experience your services and your team. Are you open to this? We've met many leaders who resist, thinking they already know what their customers want and need.

⚒ Tool: Listening-to-Customers Attitude Check

Purpose. This tool assesses your own openness to seeking out and listening to your customers' needs and perceptions.

Method. Answer true or false:

- I believe that I do know what my customers want from our services.
- Customers don't know how to express their needs and wants very clearly.
- Talking to customers takes more time than I can afford to spend.
- I've taken pains to listen to our customers before and didn't really learn much of value.
- I'm afraid to ask customers what they want, for fear that I won't be able to do what's required to meet their needs.
- I don't know how to keep the conversation focused on wants and needs rather than problems to solve.
- I don't believe that I should be the one to talk to customers.

Time to draw conclusions. The more of these statements that you answered with true, the more you are thinking like a provider-oriented manager. You think you are wasting your time listening to customers, that you already have the answers. We want to challenge these thoughts, by examining the contrasting beliefs held by the customer-obsessed manager.

When thinking about listening to customers, the customer-obsessed manager has these beliefs:

- I think I do know what our customers want, but I would like to know if I'm on target.
- Customer needs are always changing, and I have to keep asking questions to make sure that we're on the right course.
- If I learn anything at all, it will have been worth it.
- My staff needs to know that we are making changes and improvements based on what our customers are telling us. If we don't ask, we won't know.

Did you discover there are good reasons to devote time and planning to asking customers what they want, expect, and perceive regarding your services? We hope so.

There are many ways to solicit customer views: surveys, focus groups, interviews, and so on. But regardless of method, the danger is letting your own bias cloud your questions and conclusions. This next tool helps you avoid this danger by asking simple, open-ended questions and checking back with customers to make sure what you are hearing is what they are saying.

✖ Tool: Customer, What Do You Expect?

Purpose This tool asks customers what they want and expect and uses what you learn to refine your services.

Method. Talk to one customer a day for a few minutes. Good questions to ask are:

- When you call our department or office, or come to see us for service, what does it take to satisfy you?
- What does it take to make that happen? What can we do or say that would make a difference?
- What can we do not to dissatisfy you but to wow you with our service?

Do this every day for two weeks. Make sure you are talking to internal as well as external customers.

Interviewing customers with an open mind is critical. Always eye opening, it enables you to gather valuable information that leads you to do the things that reflect your customer obsession.

Another eye-opening experience is called "Walk in the Shoes." This is one of Gail's favorite tools from her Leading for Excellence Toolkit. It is a critical point in her service work, and clients have found it invaluable in helping them view their service from the customer's perspective. With this tool, we suggest that you either go through your service, experiencing it as a customer would, or be a shadow and follow a customer as this person proceeds through your service process. You will be amazed at what you can learn just by watching. Of course, you want to talk to the customers at the end to find out their perceptions, since these may be different from yours. Make sure to use the data collector provided, so you have an easy way to share your learning with your team.

⚒ Tool: Walk in the Shoes (Scott, 1997b)

Purposes. This tool helps you understand your customer's experience as he or she uses your service; it identifies opportunities for celebration and improvement.

Method. Select the customer process that you want to understand better (for instance, admitting, scheduling, procuring supplies). The goal is to create a realistic experience. You really want to "get horizontal" and see things from the customer's perspective.

Use the grid below to help you think through and capture the details of your experience.

Walk in the Shoes: Data Collector

Steps in the Process	What Was Done	What Was Said	Customer Reactions	Your Reactions	Possibilities for Change

Reflect on what you've seen, and plan a time to share this with your staff. Take care to focus on awareness of customer satisfaction. Don't judge or reprimand people for aspects of the service that were disappointing. Shape your communication as a wonderful learning opportunity.

Engage your staff as well in walking in customer shoes. By adopting a customer perspective and asking real customers what they want and what they experience, you take a giant step toward performing the actions that are the key to customer obsession.

What's next? So far, we've shared tools that can help you strengthen your focus on customers and get closer to them and what they want and need if they are to feel well served. But we know you don't operate in a vacuum. Your next challenge is to make your dedication and excitement about serving customers contagious among your staff, cultivating their customer orientation too and involving them in making service quality ever better.

Strategy Three: Engage Your Team

Begin by having staff members interview and shadow customers. You might need to do some coaching on the side as your team develops a much keener understanding of their customers, what the team is doing well for these customers, and opportunities for improvement. The good news is, if you engage your team in interviewing and observing customers to learn about their perspective, you won't need to be the exclusive salesperson for your customer obsession, because your team members will develop it themselves.

The next step is a real challenge. Assuming you learn from your customers regularly, how do you turn what you learn into constructive action of value to the customer and your organization? The answer is to make sure that everyone on the team is saying and doing what the customer needs. This next tool helps you engage your team in creating high standards (and concrete ones) related to customer expectation. Once you have interviewed and shadowed customers, using this tool is a snap.

✪ Tool: What Will It Take? (Scott, 1997c)

Purpose. This tool translates customer expectations into specific standards or behavioral expectations. It identifies opportunities for improvement in meeting these standards consistently, makes sure that behavioral expectations mean the same to everyone on the team, and develops shared ownership of high expectations.

Method. Review with your team what everyone learned in talking with customers about the service features important to them when using the service—features such as keeping the noise down, getting respect, being listened to, receiving complete information, being seen on time, and the like. Place each expectation on a flipchart sheet, and mount the pages around the room. Ask the group to create a sentence or two under *each* expectation that clarifies and expands on it.

- Break the large group into smaller groups, with one group standing in front of each flipchart. Give the small groups ten minutes to flesh out specific dos and don'ts related to the expectation on their flipchart, including examples and how-to's that reflect the work they do.

- After ten minutes, have the groups rotate to another flipchart. Ask them to look over the list done by the previous group and find ways to make the ideas more specific and more complete. They should refine the list as they see it.

- After another ten minutes, have groups rotate again to another flipchart. This time, the small groups should look at the list in front of them and think about editing it so that they push for excellence, dazzle customers, and stretch for the best they can be.

- Groups rotate one more time and give another list a final once-over with an eye to fine-tuning language, collapsing redundant information, and adding final touches. The result should be a complete list under each heading, a list that spells out what employees could and should be doing to demonstrate that behavior.

- These groups then look over their list and prepare to give a five-minute presentation about it to the large group. The goal is to explain why these new behaviors and expectations are important now and in the future.

The preceding tool is a bit challenging to facilitate, but the results are amazing. Your team fleshes out expectations in great detail, and they own them. It is important to involve as many of your team members as you can, since you want your whole team to understand and endorse the new expectations. If your organization already has explicit service expectations in place, you can apply the tool using these expectations as flipchart headers. The key for your group is to understand how service expectations relate to the work *they* do—to be quite specific and concrete. Your role is helping them understand and make that connection.

This next tool helps you advance another step in the process of moving from good to impressive, by looking at a select few service behaviors at a time. Our experience is that many managers try to impose too many expectations on their team at once. They raise awareness, but they don't see much in the way of behavior change, and they don't achieve accountability. We believe that impressive service is about the details, the little things, and you need to focus the group's attention on these details one step at a time.

✪ Tool: Moving from Good to Impressive (Leebov, Scott, and Olson, 1998)

Purpose. This tool helps staff think through ways they can move from good to impressive by identifying and fine-tuning specific behavior.

Method. Choose one behavior that you know matters to customers and that you know your team needs to improve. This could be making a great first impression, showing that we care, anticipating customer needs, explaining what we are doing, or another of importance to your specific customers.

- At a staff meeting, ask your team to think about common situations in which they have an opportunity to demonstrate the chosen behavior. Narrow this list down to a few opportunities that most people have within their jobs.

- Ask people to describe their typical behavior in these situations. Help people define what it takes to move from the typical way they demonstrate these behaviors to the *exceptional* way that would wow their customers.

- In small groups, ask the staff to look over the examples and identify one or two things that everyone could do to move from good to impressive. Have the groups share their results with everyone, and ask for group commitment to engage in these new behaviors in the coming weeks.

To reach the level of explicitness that makes it easier for your team to perform impressively in relation to customer needs, you'll need to keep the importance of customers and service quality on the front burner. After all, out of sight, out of mind. We realize that you are juggling multiple priorities, but a manager with an enduring customer obsession drives *continuous* service improvement.

To accomplish this, you need to maintain your focus and communicate it over and over, in many ways, in every meeting and forum. In fact, every time people convene, you can reinforce your customer obsession and service commitment by talking about customer needs and service priorities, sharing plans, snags, progress, and results. The three tools that follow are great examples of how you can maintain your focus and momentum with your team. The first you can use to start every meeting with a customer focus. The next two are easy ways to help your team share appreciation and recognition for delivering service valued by customers.

Tool: Quick Service Warm-Ups (Leebov, Scott, and Olson, 1998)

Purpose. This tool begins meetings with a ritual that keeps customer service primary in people's minds, while also giving your team members a lift as they proceed through their busy day and routine.

Method. Introduce a ritual of having a short five-minute warm-up activity at every meeting to help people focus on priorities.

Use service-related warm-ups that keep people thinking and talking about service. To get started, use the suggestions that follow. Then make up your own. Use one per meeting, and invite other topics or start this same list over again. By then, people will have new answers.

Introduce the warm-ups. Say, "As a warm-up, let's start by going around and having everyone complete this sentence. If you can't think of something, it's OK to pass; then at the end, you can have a turn. So, take a minute and think of what you want to say."

- Warm-up one: a compliment I got from a customer this week was ____________.
- Warm-up two: a service improvement I'm personally working on is ____________.

- Warm-up three: if I ran this service, an improvement I'd make for the sake of our customers is _____.

- Warm-up four: a tough service situation that came up for me this week was _____.

- Warm-up five: if we could hear our customers talking about us, I think we'd hear them say _____.

- Warm-up six: if our customers had a magic wand to wave and make a change in our service, I bet they would _____.

- Warm-up seven: when it comes to serving my customers, I wish I could get some help in being better at _____.

- Warm-up eight: the funniest thing that happened this week between a customer and me was _____.

- Warm-up nine: a great service interaction I noticed a coworker having was when _____.

- Warm-up ten: a time this week when someone here made it easier for me to provide good service was when _____.

Tips to make this effective:

- Participate yourself.

- Model superb listening skills as people share.

- At the end, thank people for sharing.

The next tool is another complementary approach that focuses on accomplishments and successes.

 ## Tool: Service Recognition Warm-Ups (Leebov, Scott, and Olson, 1998)

Purpose. This tool starts staff meetings in a way that helps staff recognize the positive service contributions they and their peers make.

Method. Mix these warm-ups with the quick service warm-ups just described.

- Ask, "Since we last met, what good example of great service to customers have you seen someone here provide?"

- Thank someone publicly for his or her exemplary performance and customer-oriented attitude in a specific situation that occurred recently. Tell it as a story.

- Ask people to brag about one example of great service they provided since you saw each other last.

- Commend the group on a service strength you noticed in the last week.

Next is a tool that focuses staff on successes, since success in meeting customer needs sparks further success.

✖ Tool: Success of the Week (Scott, 1997a)

Purpose. This tool focuses your team on what's going well in the way of service, to make it easy for staff to share their service successes.

Method. At the start of a staff meeting, ask people to think about a service interaction or incident that they feel good about. Give them a minute to share this interaction or incident with a partner.

- After a couple of minutes, ask people to share with the larger group what the partner did. If it's a large group, invite a few sample stories. If it's a small group, invite everyone to share the partner's story. Ask people which story they would like to select as the service success of the week. Try to reach consensus.

- Write up the success of the week and post it on a bulletin board along with a snapshot of the person the story is about. Do this yourself, or ask for a volunteer to do it.

These activities help you keep your customer obsession on the front burner. They demonstrate the obsession feature—that the importance of customers and service quality never goes away. It is always a priority. It cannot be forgotten. You can set this tone by building a customer focus ritual into an everyday activity.

With a Customer Obsession, Everyone Wins

Embracing and then holding tight to a customer obsession is not easy, especially in the fray of everyday pressure to focus on such things as service delivery, productivity, systems problems, and financial constraints and results. But the provider orientation of the past no longer works. It is the dynamic organization and the inspiring manager who recognize the incredible power of satisfying customers—a power that yields rich rewards for patients and other customers, your team members who want to take pride in their work, and you (since you want not only to earn your keep but also make a valued and respected contribution to the mission and success of your organization).

Good luck, and share your stories with us. We collect them.

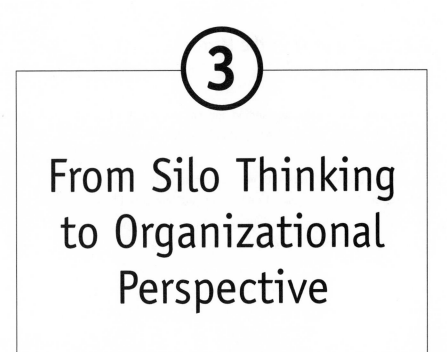

From Silo Thinking to Organizational Perspective

Your organization is grander than the sum of its parts. Its many elements interconnect and affect each other. These days, an organizational perspective is critical to tapping this potential. This means leaving the safety of the silo and crossing boundaries.

A Revealing Look in the Mirror

True or False?	True	False
1. I spend a lot of energy understanding how my part of our operation connects to and affects parts of the operation that are others' responsibility.	____	____
2. I talk about the big picture with my staff often, so they can understand where our organization is going and how they fit.	____	____
3. My colleagues in other areas would tell you that I am a good citizen in terms of being considerate of their needs and constraints.	____	____
4. When I am thinking through a change I want to make, I take pains to identify how this change will affect people and systems that are beyond my direct authority.	____	____
5. I suggest initiatives or improvements that will strengthen our organization's services, even if they have nothing to do with my direct area of responsibility.	____	____
6. When I set my priorities, I think about what's important to the organization, not just to my own area.	____	____
7. I volunteer for interdepartmental teams because I recognize that many of our most important challenges involve interdependency across functions.	____	____
8. I make sure I'm in the loop when it comes to information about our organization's initiatives and plans.	____	____
9. When I talk with staff about a change that they don't like, I work hard to represent the *why*, so that they will understand the change from an organizational perspective.	____	____
10. When I see a significant problem in someone else's area and I think they might not be aware of it, I talk to them about it.	____	____

If you answered true to most of these statements, you tend to operate beyond your particular silo and identify with the broader organization. You also tend to see challenges and opportunities from an organizational perspective. You help your staff learn the big picture. You consider other departments when you're making changes. You cross lines to solve problems. You help your staff embrace change by taking the larger view of it. You look for solutions to challenges that extend beyond your own services.

If you considered most statements to be false, you tend to engage in silo thinking. You focus your energy, effort, and leadership within your piece of the organization. Because health care organizations are complicated with many interdependent parts, you run the risk of basing your decisions and actions on tunnel vision rather than on an organizational perspective.

It's a New Day

Have you heard the ancient Hindu fable about the five blind men and an elephant? The five men surround the elephant. One touches the elephant's tale and says, "I think we have here a rope." Another feels the broad side of the elephant and claims he has here a wall. Another feels the elephant's trunk and asserts, "We have here a tree." And so on. The point is, each man experiences only one part of the elephant. None of them has a perspective on the whole elephant and how its parts fit together, serve unique functions, and make the elephant a force to reckon with.

The health care organization is like an elephant. The manager who stays in the comfort zone of his or her individual domain fails to see the whole organization in all its complexity and interrelationships. This tunnel vision creates hazards when it comes to making enlightened decisions with the interrelationships and overall purpose in mind.

What does it mean to take an organizational perspective? Your organization is greater than the sum of its parts. Its elements connect to and affect each other over time and function toward a common purpose. The word *system* derives from the ancient Greek verb *synistanai*, which means to cause to stand together.

If you define your work world as the silo you directly manage, you contribute to disconnects among the parts of your organization. Your organization then does not hang together. If you want to revamp processes or improve systems, you have to consider the whole elephant. To see the whole elephant, you must rely on others and collaborate, since the members of your organization experience different aspects of the elephant. By determined efforts to gather the big picture, you make better decisions from a broader context. You realize the ramifications and tradeoffs involved not only for your team and customers but also for the system at large.

Take a Look

These managers handle situations very differently when they approach them from the stance of silo thinking rather than an organizational perspective.

Mary Ellen

Mary Ellen has just heard about the opening of an important new service. Approaching this surprising bit of information with silo thinking, she complains, "Nobody ever tells me anything" and feels bitter that she has been left out of the loop.

Approaching this same situation from an organizational perspective, Mary Ellen realizes that she herself needs to take initiative to stay better informed about plans, news, and priorities, so that she can support them, educate her staff about them, and align her function in support of them.

Mickey and Marvin

At a cocktail party, Community Hospital's billing manager, Mickey, is introduced to Marvin, a man who, upon realizing that Mickey works for Community, launches into a series of vehement complaints about a recent experience a family member had with Community's medical care. Prone to silo thinking, Mickey reflects, *Thank goodness, this isn't my problem.* He is sympathetic and talks with Marvin about how difficult it is to meet the many needs patients bring to the hospital and the resource constraints that make it so difficult.

Taking an organizational perspective instead, Mickey feels upset. He thinks to himself, *This is my organization, and I need to do something about this!* He apologizes to Marvin for the frustrations his family suffered, and he asks if Marvin minds if he investigates further next week. When Marvin agrees, Mickey sets his mind to talk with the people involved and helps to figure out how Community might show responsiveness so impressive that this family's dissatisfaction transforms into satisfaction. Mickey takes responsibility as an ambassador for Community, and he follows up and follows through.

Jamal

Jamal is a nurse manager. He's riding the elevator along with two physicians and two unknown people, most likely visitors. He overhears one physician talking about a patient by name and mentioning the patient's condition to the other physician. Caught up in silo thinking, Jamal minds his own business. The patient is not on his unit, and he has no relationship with these physicians. The door opens and people go their separate ways. Jamal stays within his silo even as he moves through public spaces and witnesses incidents that reflect on everyone in the organization.

In contrast, acting from an organizational perspective, Jamal intervenes. Working up his courage, he says politely, "Doctor, I'm wondering if you might hold this conversation in a more private place." Seeing himself as a member of the organization's leadership team, he acts in the best interests of Community and its reputation.

Marcus

Marcus hears about the need to make deep budget cuts. Operating on behalf of his silo, he not only lobbies his boss for the staff he needs to keep functioning but also tells his boss about certain other departments that, he believes, could stand to lose some people. Marcus is intent on minimizing his own losses, regardless of the consequences for others beyond his realm. He believes he is competing for scarce resources and goes to war to get what he needs.

Operating from an organizational perspective, Marcus talks with other managers, exploring creative solutions that lead to the best results for the organization. He advances options involving give-and-take and also pushes for process improvement to free up resources without significant negative consequences. He is protective of what's best for the organization, even at the risk of losing resources for his own area. Needless to say, when Marcus is in this mode, his boss considers him a team player.

Jessie

Jessie manages nursing in a nursing home. The assistants are up in arms because they heard that nurses in the acute care division of the same health care system were slated to receive midyear salary increases. As a silo thinker, Jessie too is up in arms. She sympathizes with her nursing assistants and expresses her disgust that the system's executives allow this devaluing of her nursing assistants to happen. She is primarily concerned with maintaining morale among her team at any cost.

In contrast, taking an organizational perspective, Jessie finds out the rationale driving the RN increases in the acute care setting. She learns all she can about it, seeks out explanations of why the nursing assistants are not in line for an increase, and then communicates with her nursing assistants to help them understand. She educates them about pay at market rates. She openly discusses pay differences between groups and shows that they are market-based, not tied to people's importance. She works to build acceptance of the pay differential decisions that she knows will be a continuing fact of life in her organization. She does not complain about the decisions as misguided. She helps her team understand them from a broader context.

What Worries You?

First of all, who has time?! Perhaps you worry about the time involved in learning what you need to learn and building the relationships you require to develop an organizational perspective. You're right to think that time is required. There is no way to get around this. The question is, Is it worth it?

Can you even grasp the complexity of the whole? Recognizing the complexity of health care systems, you may be put off by this complexity and real concern about whether you could even hope to understand the factors involved in an organizational perspective.

Won't decisions be harder to make and take longer? If you stay in your silo, you only have to consider options and their consequences for your own customers, staff, and services. You can make decisions largely in the privacy of your own office, in the privacy of your own mind. If you have to consider the implications of these alternatives for others beyond your service, you will need to attend more meetings, do more homework, sell your ideas, and address people's concerns to win their cooperation. This indeed sounds exhausting and time-consuming. It also puts you at the mercy of others' reactions. You lose some degree of control and might even have to abandon your plans. In any case, you need to involve others in the decision-making process, and every step takes time.

What Do You Stand to Gain?

Alas, we wish we could explain away these concerns, but we think they are all undeniably tied to taking an organizational perspective. Is the juice worth the squeeze?

- *Silo thinking denies reality.* Health care services are complicated animals. Functions and services are interdependent. Your services can't be excellent in a vacuum. You can hide from that fact, but you can't be effective if you do. To make good decisions and to align with your organization's overall mission and strategies, you must grasp the context, and to do that you need an organizational perspective.

- *Relatively little can be accomplished in one silo alone.* Inevitably, if you limit your work to what people in your silo can accomplish, you are not doing enough. Singly owned functions are few and far between. Most important improvements involve processes and systems that cut across department lines. Your services are better, and you can make them work better, if you start by understanding interdependency and taking it into account as you identify your priorities and take steps to strengthen your services.

- *Silo thinkers become known as blockers, obstacle makers, and naysayers.* Some silo-thinking managers tell us they believe they'll create fewer problems and ward off unwanted attention if they stick to their knitting and mind their own silo's business. We think the reverse is true. Silo thinkers create problems for others. By not participating in interdisciplinary and interfunctional initiatives, they earn resentment and disrespect from executives and fellow managers who see them as failing the team and not sharing responsibility for making the whole organization work.

- *People come to trust you.* Colleagues frequently view silo-thinking managers as loose cannons, because they implement changes that affect their services without regard to the effect on practices and people beyond their narrow scope. As a result, colleagues become suspicious. If you display an organizational perspective, your colleagues are more likely to trust you, because they know you understand, consider, and respect their role, their priorities, and the effect you have on each other.

These are giant benefits. Despite the time and energy it takes to maintain an organizational perspective, your value to your organization grows exponentially as you make this shift successfully.

What Can I Do? How Can I Do It?

We suggest five strategies if you choose to make a transition from silo thinking to an organizational perspective (Exhibit 3.1).

Exhibit 3.1. Your Organizational Perspective Toolkit.

> Strategy one: Adjust your thinking.
>
> Strategy two: Learn and communicate the big picture.
>
> Strategy three: Include consciously.
>
> Strategy four: Stretch your perspective.
>
> Strategy five: Intervene on behalf of the organization.

The first strategy helps you shift further away from silo thinking than you already are. We think it helps to start by looking at your beliefs and making sure they align with an organizational perspective.

The second strategy presents tools for learning about the big picture in your organization, so that you can approach situations and decisions with an organizational perspective. It also offers tools for communicating the big picture to your team members, so they join you in this broader perspective.

A powerful way to be sure you're benefiting from an organizational perspective is to bring multiple perspectives into the room—invite into the dialogue people from other parts of the organization. Strategy number three is about "conscious inclusion"—consciously and conscientiously drawing others into a situation where you and your team can benefit from their knowledge, issues, and viewpoints.

The fourth strategy is about mind stretching. We present analytical tools you can use to push yourself to think organization, not silo. By asking yourself the right questions, you can develop a habit of thinking about the consequences for others beyond the domain of decisions you face.

The final strategy requires some boldness on your part. It calls for intervening when you are witness to a situation where the organization's best interests are not being advanced.

Strategy One: Adjust Your Thinking

Perhaps you have concerns about adopting an organizational perspective, and they dissuade you from making the shift. This first tool helps you consider and address your concerns.

⚒ Tool: Write and Debate

Purpose. This tool identifies your concerns about adopting an organizational perspective and helps the wise person in you allay these concerns.

Method. Begin by writing nonstop. Abandon all inhibition and write down as fast as you can every feeling, thought, and concern you have about collaborating with other people across department, service, or divisional lines. Do this for three minutes (using an egg timer if you have one handy). Then read and reread what you've written.

Now debate the other side of the matter. Push yourself to think like a manager who already has a strong organizational perspective. Jot down the main points this manager would make to debate the feelings, concerns, and thoughts that discourage you from collaborating with others across lines (see example below).

Write and Debate: An Example

Excerpt from one manager's nonstop writing

I'm afraid others will see what I'm doing and think of me as incompetent.

I'm afraid others will make more demands on me or question my priorities.

I'm concerned that I will have to work with Melvin, whom I've been able to ignore up to now.

The manager's response

You're kidding yourself. You're not really doing a good job when you hide in your silo. Other people see that and they respect you less for it.

The wise person within you knows why an organizational perspective is essential in today's environment. Tap into this wise person to address your own resistance and reorient your thinking to support breaking out of your silo once and for all.

Once you have your thoughts under control, it's time for action that broadens your perspective with rich information, to help you grasp the complexity of your environment and services and the interdependency of the parts on each other.

Strategy Two: Learn and Communicate the Big Picture

Can you draw the big picture of the organization's main strategies for the next two years? Can you explain this to a friend?

If so, great! Your awareness and retention of this plan demonstrate an organizational perspective. If not, you may be so absorbed with operations in your area that you are disconnected from the broader context. To move out of what is in this case an information silo, take the initiative to get the information critical to articulating this plan, or at least the main strategies your organization is engaged in at this time.

Here are two tools to help you learn the big picture.

✖ Tool: Big-Picture Interview

Purpose. This tool puts you in the know by asking questions of someone else who is in the information loop.

Method. Identify one or two people whom you perceive to be in the loop of information about where your organization is going.

- Call or e-mail them, asking them if they would join you for lunch or agree to an appointment. Tell them you would like to interview them because you want to learn more about where the organization is going and you value their perspective.

- Set a time for the interview or lunch and ask them these questions, being sure to listen well and take notes.

Questions: Where Are We Going?

1. What do you see as the main challenges our organization faces in the next two years?

2. How are we doing in the face of these challenges?

3. In the face of these challenges, what are we doing not only to survive but also to thrive in pursuit of our mission?

4. What do you see as our main strengths that will help us become or remain successful?

5. As you know, I'm responsible for the _____ department. How do you see my department contributing to our success strategies? What do you see as our important roles?

What's the point? Go after the information you want and need, instead of waiting for others to tell you what you must know. They might never think to do that, and then you are left in the lurch uninformed and probably resentful. Act first. Ask for reports to read; arrange interviews. Assertively ask to be kept in the loop on initiatives that you feel you should understand.

Another idea is to create a support system for yourself to help you connect to other managers and learn about the complexities of organizational strategy and organizational life in discussions with them. Talk about:

- Plans that you are working on
- Changes you are considering
- Problems you are facing
- Successes you are having

Seeking information, seeing your function and others' from multiple angles, connecting with customers and other managers, asking questions, reading everything that crosses your desk even if it has seemingly nothing to do with your immediate priorities—all of these activities help you gain the sense of context that helps you integrate your work and your team with the work of the organization, thereby maximizing your contribution.

You aren't the only one who needs to stay informed; your staff must feel in the know as well. Consider the next tool as a way your boss can augment and reinforce big-picture thinking among your team.

⚒ Tool: Skip-Level Meetings

Purpose. This tool expands your team's understanding of the organization's mission, vision, values, goals, and strategies so that they feel in the know, and so they better understand how they fit in the organization.

Method. Each quarter, invite your boss to join you and your staff for a meeting. Before the meeting, solicit questions from your staff as to "things we want to know about our organization." Make sure you include your questions too. Give your boss the list of questions a week ahead of time, so as not to blind-side your boss.

Hold the meeting and reinforce how important it is to you for your team to stay in the know so they can contribute to the organization's strategy and progress.

This approach helps bridge the communication gap and has an added benefit of helping to eliminate the us-versus-them feelings that exist in so many organizations, by bringing staff and administrators together. Result? Organizational understanding on many levels. Our next strategy takes the concept of pulling people from other silos into your domain one step further.

Strategy Three: Include Consciously

Think about a decision that someone else made without consulting you, one that had an adverse affect on you and your group. How did it feel? What do you wish this individual or group had done differently? How often does this happen in your organization?

In many organizations, this type of situation happens every day, with negative consequences for customers and staff—not to mention the time it sometimes takes to undo the decisions. What to do?

Changing this dynamic won't be easy, but it begins with becoming more conscious of whom to include when you hold meetings to plan, solve problems, allocate work and resources, and communicate. Ask yourself the questions in the next tool, and we know that you will be able to identify people who are instrumental or affected by your plans. By using this tool, you can consciously decide whether they should be involved and whether to involve them sooner or later.

✖ Tool: Meeting Mix Memory Aid

Purpose. This tool helps you consciously decide whom to include in meetings, when you're intent on acting for the good of the whole.

Method. Think "intra" to identify people within your organization, think "inter" to identify people from other organizations within your system, and think "external" to include people outside of your system whom it is also appropriate to involve. Ask:

- Who is affected? Whose areas and people are affected?
- Who can help us move quickly and well?
- Who is it important to involve now, so we are all aligned down the road?
- Who will we need in order to pull this off?

- Who will have or share responsibility for the results and plans that come from the discussion, such that they should be involved early on?

- Who has an important perspective to add to our discussion, resulting in better decisions?

Strategy Four: Stretch Your Perspective

It is difficult to demonstrate an organizational perspective if you don't, despite your intentions, see relationships and interconnections. In fact, if you don't understand how the work you do relates to the work that everyone else does, you won't even think to consider them in plans and meetings. Yet to see them as partners requires more than motivation. It also requires analytical skill. The tools in this next section help you focus your analytical skills to stretch your perspective.

Tool: Mapping Downstream and Upstream Consequences

Purpose. This tool helps you think through and portray the precursors and consequences of your decisions and plans, demonstrating your concern about the impact of your services and plans on others beyond your scope.

Method. When you're making a decision, go beyond examining how solutions solve the problem within your direct line of sight. Use mapping to consider the consequences (see sample below).

Checking Consequences: An Example

A rehab unit decides it has the potential to attract many more patients to its sports medicine outpatient services. The leadership team figures out a revenue target and realizes that they have marketing strategies available to them that can help them meet or exceed that target:

- Before going full speed ahead, taking an organizational perspective, they ask themselves, *If we increase our volume in that program, who else beyond our outpatient service site will be affected?*

- Will nonstaff orthopedists lose volume if we increase it?

- Since more outpatient volume will increase surgery business, do our surgeons have the capacity to handle more volume?

- If our surgeons do have the capacity to handle more volume, does our OR schedule have the capacity to accommodate more cases from these surgeons?

- After identifying all of the groups and individuals affected by the decision, before you proceed to implement it, bring these people together to discuss your proposed plans and explore the consequences with them. As a manager with an organizational perspective, you really don't have a plan until you work out the kinks and opportunities that extend way beyond your silo of activity.

On a sheet of paper, draw a circle with your solution in it. Ask yourself what the consequences would be if you were to implement this solution. Write these consequences in circles leading from your original circle. Then, identify the consequences of each consequence, creating a map of consequences (see sample below).

Map of Consequences

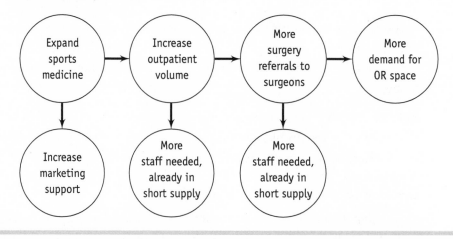

This kind of mapping helps especially when considering a decision or plan. Our next tool helps you adopt an organizational perspective when you are addressing a *problem*. This is particularly important as many managers are prone to silo thinking when they have a problem or when something goes wrong. The first instinct is to look for someone to blame, preferably someone in another silo. This enables the manager to bow out of problem solving, thinking, *It isn't our fault,* or *It's not my job,* or *It's not my department.* Some managers do seek solutions, but only within their own departments. This is tempting, because you have more control here. The problem is, most problems do not restrict themselves to one silo. They cross into others, especially if you're intent on tackling problems at their root instead of at the symptom level.

If you are prone to these patterns, try using this next tool as a simple way to unhook from a tendency to blame and restrict solutions to what you yourself can control.

⚙ Tool: The Five-*Whys* Path out of Your Silo

Purpose. This tool stops you from blaming others for problems and helps you seek root causes in the *systems or processes* that produced those problems, whether they are within or beyond your silo.

Method. Establish one ground rule: "people" cannot be the answer. We are not allowed to name people, or even attribute these symptoms to people. Let's assume that *systems* created the problem, not people.

Pick the symptom of a problem you want to tackle. Focus your group on it. Ask your first *why*: "Why is this happening?" You'll get a few answers. Post them on a flipchart or wallboard.

For each statement you've posted, ask why again: "Why is this?" Write the answers nearby.

Do this three more times (resulting in five *whys*). Then look at the answers, inviting your group to look for patterns. Typically, a five-*why* analysis converges on one or two root causes of the problem. All roads lead back to Rome. Here is an illustration.

An Example of the Five *Whys*

Symptom: An outpatient is angry because of a very long wait in radiology.

Why number one: The radiology receptionist was not there when the patient arrived.

Why number two: The patient was given an appointment time earlier than the starting time of the receptionist.

Why number three: Patients are frequently late. By making a practice of telling patients to get there early, they are more likely to be on time.

Why number four: Patient compliance is low, causing patients to be late or not show at all.

Why number five: Patients get nervous and uncertain—about what the appointment will entail, what the results will show, where to park, where to go, what to wear, and much more.

The five *whys* lead you to root causes, inevitably going beyond your department's lines. In this example, the five *whys* led to identification of the root cause of much patient lateness or missed appointments as patient anxiety—anxiety about the procedure, the results, and how to find their way. Who are all the people who can influence that?

- The patient's physician

- The technologist, who could communicate more about the test before-hand

- The marketing person, who could produce clean instructions about how to find Radiology and other outpatient areas

- The patient education coordinator

- The supervisor in Radiology, who could arrange for a system of reminder phone calls to patients the evening before their appointment

- Information Services, which has recently benchmarked a patient scheduling system that works for both staff and patients

The five *whys* lead you to root causes that typically involve areas beyond yours. You can then identify the set of people with a stake and role in addressing the problem, those with an organizational perspective built into the group.

The next strategy we want to share addresses the role of your personal behavior, specifically your assertiveness when an organizational perspective is *missing* from a situation and you have the opportunity to intervene.

Strategy Five: Intervene on Behalf of the Organization

It's one thing to see the connections between the various parts of your organization. It's another to act on these connections—to actively take responsibility, to look out for your partners and colleagues and their customers, to act as though you are an owner with a stake in the organization's overall success.

Owners don't want problems to go unsolved; they do what it takes to fix what can be fixed. They don't think *This isn't my job.* They think *This is my organization.*

Owners don't want customers to be unhappy. They take customers and their concerns seriously, even when unrelated to their specific service. If they can't solve a problem personally, they find someone who can, even if it takes phone calls, e-mails, and follow-up. Owners think, *Our customers belong to all of us.*

Owners care about everyone who works for the organization, not only about their own direct reports. Owners think, *We are this organization.*

People who think and act like owners see opportunity every day to act with an organizational perspective. But this isn't easy. It means stepping out of your comfort zone, taking the time to get involved, and at times risking disapproval from others who might prefer that you mind your own business.

When you see an issue that goes beyond your direct span of influence, you have four main options, each alternative producing its own outcome. Your challenge is to choose the appropriate option given the situation (Exhibit 3.2).

Exhibit 3.2. Alternative Ways to Intervene on Behalf of the Organization.

1. Do nothing.

2. Tell someone about the situation.

3. Report it and make sure someone handles it.

4. Offer help and assistance to solve the problem.

This next tool presents a few situations. We ask you to practice applying your organizational perspective by considering each situation, deciding how you would intervene and the consequences of your behavior.

⚒ Tool: Exploring Your Options in an Everyday Situation

Purpose. This tool considers how you can act on behalf of the organization, thus sharing responsibility.

Method. Think about the situations in Exhibit 3.3. Check the action you would normally choose and the consequences of this action.

Exhibit 3.3. A Push Toward Organizational Perspective.

Situation	Your Current Actions	Consequences	An Alternative from an Organizational Perspective	Benefits to You and Others
You walk by a patient room and see a call light on. You don't work on this unit.				
You see trash in a public area. You're late for a meeting.				
You are getting ready for a public gathering. You notice that the main hallway is littered with broken chairs. You realize this makes a negative impression.				
At a gathering, someone complains to you about the care in another part of your organization.				
At a professional meeting, you overhear people sharing false information about the organization.				
You overhear employees talking negatively about another department.				

Identify whether you are already operating from an organizational perspective. If not, think about how you could act differently, and identify the outcomes of that.

The more you operate from an organizational perspective, the more often you choose to intervene in a situation of this sort, taking responsibility to produce the best possible results.

Some of these and other situations drawing on an organizational perspective require you to be the bearer of bad news. Most people aren't eager to be the messenger in this situation and sometimes look to avoid it at all costs. When managers share their fears with us, they seem most concerned about retaliation, alienating others, or making matters worse by intervening. This is understandable, but we think there are ways to lessen this risk, if you learn the art of sharing bad news (Exhibit 3.4).

This last strategy shines the light on the commitment that you and your colleagues have to work as one team, crossing boundaries and acting in the best interests of the organization even if the consequences for your silo are problematic.

There are so many aspects to an organizational perspective—your mind-set and belief system, your information base, your analytical skills, and your personal behaviors.

You Can't Add Value Without It

An organizational perspective is not for the faint of heart. To embrace an organizational perspective, you need courage, because your plans, problems, accomplishments, and personal behaviors become visible. You place yourself in a position of accountability to your colleagues and the organization as a whole. Yet your job these days is all about adding value. To add value, you have to understand the big picture, share this understanding with your team, and craft your priorities and plans with the big picture and the organization's interests in mind.

Exhibit 3.4. Tips for Tough Communications.

- *Share your intentions.* People are less anxious when they know what to expect. For example, "I want to improve my relationship with you."

- *Put yourself in the other person's shoes.* Think about how you would feel. Watch what you say and how you say it, so you don't come across as judgmental or superior ("I understand there may be several sides to this story, and I only heard one piece, but I thought it would be helpful for you to hear this feedback from me").

- *Be specific and descriptive.* People want the details. Keep it simple. Say what you heard; don't edit or interpret. For example, "This woman said she had to wait for a very long time, more than an hour, and that no one stopped to explain why she was waiting. She said when she asked questions, staff rolled their eyes and made her feel as though she was a bother. She was frustrated and said that she didn't intend to use us and our services again."

- *Show empathy.* People are less defensive if they think you understand. Put yourself in their shoes. Think about what it might feel like from their point of view ("I know we're all very busy. This complaint could have been directed to any of us on any given day. I can imagine that your staff was responding out of their own frustration").

- *Offer support or assistance.* Make sure you let the person know that you are willing to help if you can ("I also know that we all need to work with our teams so they understand our goals of achieving impressive service. Is there anything I can do to help you?").

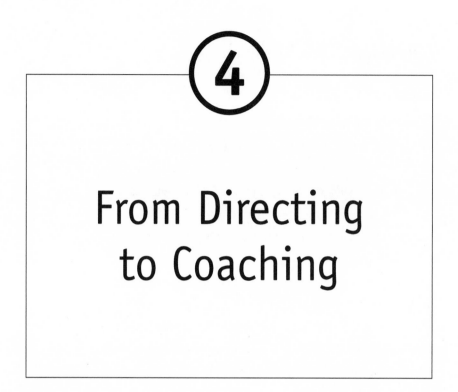

From Directing
to Coaching

The directing style of management will always have its place, but today it needs to take a backseat to coaching. Workteams benefit from coaching as much as athletic teams do. Managers need to become coaches; they too can create champions.

A Revealing Look in the Mirror

True or False?	True	False
1. I recognize and reward learning among my team.	____	____
2. I know that my people have a great deal of potential and rely on me to help them develop.	____	____
3. I am always looking for new ways to motivate and energize my team.	____	____
4. I devote time to getting to know my staff personally and professionally.	____	____
5. I match work assignments with the skills and interests of individuals on my team.	____	____
6. When I am pressed for time, I find it is easier to just do the task, rather than delegate it.	____	____
7. When people make mistakes, I tend to avoid asking them to do other things in the future.	____	____
8. I am very frustrated when my staff members don't do things the way I believe they should be done.	____	____
9. I am not comfortable dealing with performance issues.	____	____
10. My staff have difficulty getting access to me.	____	____

If you answered true to the first five questions and false to the remaining five, you are thinking and acting more like a coach than a director. Good coaches devote time to helping people develop their capabilities. They recognize the importance of their coaching to the people they coach. They take steps to get to know people personally and professionally, so they can tailor tasks and learning opportunities to them. Also, a good coach avoids jumping in to complete a task when the person being coached is floundering. Instead, the coach offers feedback and support.

For some managers, coaching comes naturally, but many of us have to work hard to shift from directing to coaching. For one thing, many of us learned a director style from our early role models. Many of our teachers, scout leaders, and even our (literal) coaches exhibited this style of leadership. Thus many of us learned at an early age that directing is the appropriate way to behave when in a position of authority.

Also, many people who end up in a management position have a directive or authoritative personality style. We want things done a certain way and have difficulty letting go of control unless we feel confident that the outcomes will meet our requirements. We often find it easier or more comfortable to just do it ourselves than to help someone else learn how.

It's a New Day

Several forces in today's environment compel us to become a skilled *coach* rather than a director. First, there's too much work to do to get it all done alone. It is just too big a job. Many managers we know tell us they feel they're drowning in work. When we raise the option of delegating some of their tasks, they roll their eyes and say, "Are you kidding? I have nobody who can do the job. It's easier to do it myself." Their work piles up, with no hope for relief.

The shift to a coaching style is also important because of our employees' expectations and needs. Employees today want their leaders to take an interest in them and help them develop their skills and abilities. They expect to be included in decision making. Most are uncomfortable being repeatedly told what to do.

What does this mean for you? You walk a tightrope. Organizations need leaders who are decisive and can call the shots and take charge. At the same time and paradoxically, they need leaders who can create a work environment where people are self-managing, independently resourceful, and autonomous.

You must navigate both roles and understand how and when to use each role to get the work done and the results you seek. But referring back to tradition and longstanding patterns, this is especially hard because most leaders we know find much greater comfort in the director role than in the role of coach.

Take a Look

Meet three managers in situations facing them, to see the difference between a directing and a coaching approach.

Todd

Todd has recently taken over a large service department. Within the system, the department has a reputation of being weak. He sees many changes he wants to make related to cost reduction as well as service improvement. If he is not successful at both goals, the organization will probably outsource his service. Todd's hiring reflects a last-ditch effort on the part of administration to keep the function in-house.

The members of Todd's staff have been used to an old-style leader who just told them what to do. Most are not used to thinking for themselves and are uncomfortable when expected to take initiative or otherwise act empowered. However, quite a few department members do have what it takes to help lead the team, and these people could be a great asset in engaging their coworkers in improving the department's performance.

Many managers would probably view Todd's situation as hopeless and dread having to make the changes that he faces. Others might see that change is a must and proceed to develop a plan on their own, implementing the changes by just telling the team what to do.

A manager comfortable with a coach or mentor role views this situation as an opportunity to develop the team and individual talent, as well as an opportunity to improve the department's services. This leader engages staff in creating a shared vision for the department and helps the group understand where they fit into this new vision.

If there are tasks that need to be completed and jobs that need to be designed, the coaching leader tries to match these tasks and responsibilities to the skills and interests of team members.

Rosita

Rosita is the head of a large marketing department. She is responsible for all of the internal and external communications in the system, as well as for public and community relations. She has several supervisors reporting to her, but she is having difficulty getting this group to run with the ball. They seem to come to her with everything and disappoint her by not making decisions on their own.

As a directing manager, Rosita rationalizes that this is just the way these folks are. She issues directives that they seem to need and does nothing to change the situation. Sometimes, in her frustration, she gets upset with the group and shares her disappointment with them, making people feel even more inadequate.

Acting instead as a coach, Rosita responds differently. She understands her responsibility for changing the dynamics among her team. Although it requires time and effort, she knows she needs to work with each person individually to bring out the best. Rosita looks at her own behavior to see what she does that creates uneasiness and lack of confidence among her staff.

Helen

Helen has two team members who need a great deal of attention. Their skills are insufficient, and they each have emotional or family problems that make it hard for them to focus on their work. These are, however, long-term employees. Helen knows that replacing these individuals will not be easy.

As a directing manager, Helen tries to work around the problems, suspecting that she will have to ultimately replace both employees. Others on the team resent Helen for giving them more work to compensate for what the two problem employees are failing to do.

As a coaching manager, Helen considers other options. She investigates support resources available within her organization, including the employee assistance program, Human Resources' employee relations specialist, and the training department. She seeks to find out which counseling or training options could help these employees address the personal issues affecting their job performance. She also talks with colleagues about who on the team might serve as a buddy for the employees, helping them improve their job skills.

As a coaching manager, Helen understands that she can't be all things to all people, that her job is to do what she can to get people the help they need if possible and point them in the right direction.

As coaching managers, Todd, Rosita, and Helen all devote considerable time to developing their teams. But many managers fear that taking on the role of coach is just too time-consuming. Let's take a look at this and other concerns that might also be standing in your way, as you consider directing less and coaching more.

What Worries You?

Are you afraid coaching will eat away at your already precious time? It *is* often faster and easier to do the job yourself. In today's pressure-cooker environment, it is hard to consider options that take more time, when you are already stretched to the max. But of course, you then drown in work that you're doing, while other people aren't doing theirs.

Do you think some employees just want you to tell them what to do? You may be concerned that some staff members will resist coaching and the responsibility it entails for them because they just prefer that you give them directives and answers. They have been brought up this way, and they expect you to just tell them what to do.

Are you afraid of losing control? Certainly, there are times when you will want to and need to don your director hat. You may be concerned that if you move too far toward coaching, people will no longer respond when you are more authoritative and assertive.

Are you worried that you cannot effectively coach people, given individual differences in styles, needs, and talents? Knowing that people differ and have various needs, many leaders lack confidence that they can coach effectively, given these differences within their team.

Are you afraid that employees with greater responsibility will make mistakes, and you'll receive the blame? The bottom line is that you are accountable. The buck does stop with you. Many leaders are uncomfortable letting go because they don't think the group will do the job the way it needs to be done, leaving them to take the consequences.

Do you like people's dependence on you and not want to risk losing that? Many managers like having the answers and being needed. They enjoy the thought, *If it weren't for me, things would fall apart.* This supports the need to feel important and valued. Some worry that they might lose this feeling if they rely more on their employees and the employees perform successfully.

Are you afraid you'll make yourself obsolete? Some managers are afraid of no longer being needed. They worry that they might be replaced if their staff become as capable and skilled as they are.

Since concerns about losing control and no longer being needed arise for managers crossing the bridge from director to coach, crossing it can be an uphill battle. If you have achieved comfort with a directive style, learning to be a coach definitely takes work.

What Do You Stand to Gain?

Although the concerns we have cited might deter you from shifting to more of a coach role, we know there are many benefits to making this shift.

- *You'll have happier employees.* When people learn, take on more challenging work, and receive coaching to do it well, they feel better about themselves and their abilities, and they feel better about you and the work environment.
- *You'll have employees who contribute more.* Most people are not using their full potential. Imagine what it could be like to unleash the as-yet untapped talent that exists in your group.
- *You'll gain satisfaction from the role of coach and mentor.* It can feel great to be a catalyst for someone's growth and development. Picture the times you have turned someone around. Didn't you feel as though you really made a difference? Helping your team develop is a way of giving back for the investment your own coaches and role models made in you.
- *Miracle worker though you are, you cannot do all the work there is to do.* You can't do it all yourself. Think about how different your job and your own work-life balance would be if you had a team of peak performers.
- *Coaching presents a growth opportunity for you.* Organizational leaders and the employee workforce alike value coaching as a critical, even pivotal management skill. By developing yourself as a coach, you are viewed as a more effective leader, and you become more marketable and employable.
- *Your employees' effectiveness makes you look good.* You gain the respect of other people in your team and organization. People notice that you are doing something right when you have a group of employees who are a positive force. Every bit of value added by your staff is value for which you receive credit.
- *Employees are itching to learn and grow, and coaching is a teaching process.* Learning opportunities are at the top of employees' reasons for staying with an organization. This is particularly true for younger workers who want to expand their skills and experience. When you serve as coach, you are helping your employees learn. They appreciate this and are likely to stay.

Without a doubt, you have much to gain both personally and professionally by directing less and coaching more. Admittedly, it is not an easy journey, since this shift upsets some long-standing patterns and takes time. Still, consider it a significant investment in the future. The time and energy you invest in helping your people now will have an enormous payoff later as your team handles more responsibility more effectively. You can achieve more balance in your life, while producing greater value to your organization.

What Can You Do? How Can You Do It?

We recommend four strategies to help you become a great coach (Exhibit 4.1).

Exhibit 4.1. Your Coaching Toolkit.

> Strategy one: Crystallize your resolve and think like a coach.
>
> Strategy two: Get to know your people as individuals.
>
> Strategy three: Set your people up for success.
>
> Strategy four: Create opportunities for learning and course correction.

The first strategy helps you crystallize your motivation to become an effective coach by considering the powerful effects one of your coaches had on you during your lifetime. It also helps you evaluate your thinking patterns to ensure that your thoughts support you as you shift toward frequent and effective coaching.

The second strategy helps you get to know each member of your team, and his or her strengths, goals, hopes, and fears. A great coach, after all, gets to know staff members well, to tailor tasks and coaching style to each individual's needs and preferences.

The third strategy helps you set up coaching situations so that the person you're coaching is likely to succeed, building both their competence and their confidence. Great coaches empower, knowing that their team members can do and accomplish much more than they think they can.

Our fourth strategy helps you to provide constructive support and feedback. Great coaches give people the opportunity to grow and stretch, helping to remove roadblocks and providing constructive, timely feedback along the way. Through it all, they avoid giving answers. They help their folks discover and institute solutions.

Strategy One: Crystallize Your Resolve and Think Like a Coach

Imagine where you would be if someone hadn't invested in you, coaching you to develop your strengths and achieve goals important to you. This first tool helps you get in touch with the powerful importance of coaching by revisiting your own experience with coaches and mentors who have had an impact on your life. By realizing the amazing power such people have had on your life, you will hopefully feel a surge of motivation to develop yourself as a coach.

Tool: Think of a Coach

Purpose. This tool ignites your motivation to become an effective coach by reminding you of a coach important to you in your own life.

Method. Go to a quiet place where you can be alone for at least fifteen minutes. Put on some soft music; turn off your phones and beepers. Make sure you are relaxed and have shut out any distracting thoughts.

Identify a person who has had an impact on your life as a coach or mentor, someone who cared about you, saw the good in you, possibly the good that you couldn't even see in yourself. This person could be a coach literally or a teacher, supervisor, relative, or friend.

Picture this person. What does he or she look like? Now picture yourself with this person. Where are you? How does it feel to be with this person who cares about you and sees what you can be?

What does this person do or say to let you know how he or she feels about you? How do you feel when you hear these feelings?

Picture this person asking you to do something challenging. You may even think, *I could never do this.* How does this person help you feel *Maybe I can*?

How does it feel to go to this person for help and support? What does the person say and do to keep you going in a good direction?

How does this person let you know you did a good job—that you succeeded and deserve to feel successful?

When you make a mistake, how does this person let you know? How does the person share constructive criticism in a way that helps you learn and grow?

What else did you learn from this person about yourself and your abilities?

Now take a few minutes to answer these questions:

- What did this person do to bring out the best in you?
- What did this person do or say to help you feel good about yourself and your abilities?
- What were the most important lessons you learned from this person?

Most of us have had one or more people in our lives who offered us invaluable coaching and helped us build our capability and confidence. Now, it's our turn. We have a tremendous opportunity in our management roles to serve this vital function for members of our team, to the benefit of each special individual, patients, and the organization.

Assuming you are eager to move forward with this shift, the next step is to ensure that you approach coaching with a mind-set that supports you in that role. This entails thinking less like a director and authority figure and more like a coach. In our experience of helping health care managers become effective coaches, we've seen that managers who turn out to be effective hold certain beliefs quite different from those held by managers who are less effective. Let's take a look at the difference.

The director believes that people want to be told what to do. Leaders with a director mind-set honestly believe that their staff members are more comfortable when just told what to do, when given clear instructions and answers. These leaders may even identify with these feelings and expect the same clear direction from their boss. In contrast, the coach believes, "People want to get involved and take on challenges, but they don't want to fail." Directors understand that sometimes employees *act* as though they want to be told what to do, because they don't trust their managers to help them succeed. If employees expect you to challenge or punish them if they make a mistake, they will play it safe, saying "Just tell me what to do."

The director believes that "the buck stops here, so I'll have to do it." Accountability weighs heavily on most of us, but this doesn't mean we have to do everything ourselves. Managers who think they need to do the work end up overworked and frantic, and their team members read the managers accurately, perceiving them to be saying, "I have to do everything, because I don't have faith in my team." In contrast, the coach believes "I can't do it all, and I don't need to." Coaches realize that they can accomplish much more if people on the team are engaged and contributing.

The director believes "I can't afford to let mistakes happen." Directing managers worry about how others view them; they don't want to look ineffective in the eyes of others. Also, they may not be comfortable with mistakes and may fear repercussions. In any case, they are not willing to risk relying on team members to do important work. In contrast, the coach believes, "Mistakes are important learning experiences." They expect mistakes and respect their power in helping people learn and grow. These leaders have a live-and-learn attitude and help their folks profit from these experiences.

The director believes that "these people don't have what it takes." Directors get frustrated at discovering gaps in people's abilities or attitudes that fly in the face of reliable performance. They think, *People either have it or they don't.* The directing manager believes that there is very little they can do to change or improve how their people think about themselves or do their work. In contrast, the coach believes "my team members have a great deal of untapped potential." Coaches see value and goodness in everyone and seek to unleash this potential. They also recognize that when people feel good about themselves, their abilities, and their accomplishments, this prods them to want to grow and develop even more.

Now reflect. Which beliefs do you identify with most? Do you find yourself thinking more like a director or a coach? What effect is this having on your behavior? What would you prefer to think?

⚒ Tool: Check Your Beliefs

Purpose. This tool helps you reflect on your own beliefs and the extent to which they encourage you to coach rather than direct.

Method. Take a look below at some differing beliefs held by coaches and directing managers.

Do You Think Like a Director or a Coach?

Directing Managers Believe:	Consequences	Coaching Managers Believe:
People want to be told.	I give instructions. I don't ask for feedback and opinions. People feel unimportant.	People want to get involved and take on challenges, but they don't want to fail.
The buck stops here, so I'll have to do it.	I don't use the talent in the team. I try to do more than I can accomplish. I wear out.	I can't do it all, and I don't need to.
I can't afford to let mistakes happen.	I worry about the outcomes. Mistakes happen, because I am overloaded. People don't get an opportunity to learn and grow.	Mistakes are important learning experiences.
These people don't have what it takes.	I don't give others a chance to learn and grow. Good people leave.	My team members have a great deal of untapped potential.

Once you have convinced yourself that coaching is a role you want to strengthen, you enter the zone of behavior and skill. What does a coach actually do? If you have read books or attended workshops on coaching, you have probably received hundreds of tips about the many skills involved in effective coaching. Drawing on our experience in helping managers become effective coaches, we are now going to share with you tools that help you get started *doing* the things that effective coaches do, starting with getting to know your staff as individuals.

Strategy Two: Get to Know Your People as Individuals

When we ask people to think about the coaches they have known, they invariably talk about the ability these coaches have to connect with a range of people. A great coach understands that people differ and have unique needs; a great coach takes steps to get to know their people, understand their different needs and hopes, and build on their strengths.

What did your coaches do to get to know you? Most likely they spent time talking to you, asking questions, and observing you in various situations. Do you spend time with your people? Do you ask probing questions to get to know them better? Here are tools to help you do just that. The first tool helps you find out how your people feel about their work right now, what they like and what they would like to change. The second tool has a different focus. It helps you identify the skills, experiences, attitudes, interests, and goals individuals bring to the job. These are wonderful conversation starters, so think about how you might use either of these tools with your team members.

The great news is that, once you get to know your people in greater depth as individuals, you automatically move toward a coaching relationship with them. You have in your mind their strengths, goals, hopes, and needs, which influence your decision making when it comes to delegating work, asking for help, forming project teams, and building learning experiences for your people—all critical coaching opportunities.

⚒ Tool: How Do You Feel About Your Job?

Purpose. This tool helps you find out how individuals on your team feel about their jobs and identify how you can help them feel even more successful.

Method. Look over these questions and select those that most expand your knowledge of your staff:

- Describe how you feel about your job right now.

- What do you like most about the work you are doing?

- What is there about your current work that you don't like much?

- How is your job good for you?

- How might your job not be good for you?

- What do you find easy to do in your job? What do you feel especially good at?

- What do you feel you're not so good at? What would you like to learn to do better?

- If you could change or improve anything about your job or your work, what would it be?

Decide how you can introduce this interview with staff. One approach is to say directly, "This team is full of talented people. I want to know people better, so I can tailor your responsibilities to your strengths and also help you learn and grow." You may feel awkward at first, but we know you will gain valuable information. Create a schedule to interview one staff member at a time, select one person a week to interview, or set aside a whole morning and set up a stream of interview appointments. Then do it, and you'll find that you learn a lot you didn't already know and that you have a better sense of possible directions you might pursue as a coach with each person.

Our next tool taps into other information, also helping you to be better able to consider appropriate responsibilities, projects, and coaching relationships tailored to each person. This tool is helpful in career coaching as well.

✨ Tool: What Do You Bring?

Purpose. This tool helps you get close to your people and discover what makes them tick.

Method. Ask individuals on your team to consider these topics, and have a discussion with them on the basis of their answers:

- Talents: What are some of the personal skills and assets that you bring to this job? What do you do well and want to build on?

- Passion: What are some things that you care about at work or outside? What gets you excited? What are you eager to learn more about?

- Experience: What have you done or experienced in the past that could help our team or group? What life experience do you have that you know could be valuable?

- Baggage: What are some things you are holding on to from your past that you think could hold you back unless you let go of them?

- Challenges: What are some opportunities you would like to explore? Are there areas you want to work on or develop?

- Future: If there were no obstacles, nothing in your way, where would you love to see yourself in five years? What would you want to do right now, within this job, to help move in that direction?

At the end of each interview, reflect on what you learn about each person and identify two or three ideas that you think could help him or her move in a positive and appropriate direction, one that is good for the person individually as well as for the organization.

It is also important to find out how your people feel about the work environment and their relationship with you, their boss. A great coach understands that helping someone grow and develop involves establishing a relationship. The more information you have about how your people like to be supported, the easier it is for you to build on their strengths and bolster their weaknesses. Here is a positive way to help you clarify these issues.

⚒ Tool: A Recent Success

Purpose. This tool helps you understand what it is that people feel has helped them be successful in the past.

Method. Ask the individual to think about a recent success. Here's a good introduction: "There are times in our careers when we feel really good about what we're doing and contributing. Think about a time when you felt you were at your best. This could involve an experience with a customer or a coworker. The key thing is that you felt tremendous energy and confidence."

Ask the person to tell the story of this success and talk about behavior and feelings, and what the person takes pride in now about that experience. Ask:

- What was the situation?
- What did you do to be successful?
- What was the outcome?
- How did you feel about yourself and your work as a result of this experience?
- Outside of yourself, what do you think contributed to your success? What supported you in the process?
- How is this situation like or unlike other situations at work?
- What are some things I might do to help you have more successful experiences in this job?

Thank the person for sharing this with you, mentioning specifically a couple of things that particularly impressed you as you listened.

The final technique in this section is quite different and a favorite of ours, because it focuses on individual differences in work and style. Since you are more or less in the role of coach at all times, this information helps you consider ways you can tailor your communications and expectations to better pull for the individual's preferred modes of operating.

⚒ Tool: What Do You Need?

Purpose. This tool helps you consider the individual's work and style preferences in your coaching relationship.

Method. Interview each person about preferences in how you relate to the person in your role as coach:

- Meetings: How often do you like to meet with your boss when you are working on a project?
- Communication: How do you like to be communicated with? E-mail, weekly face-to-face meetings, phone calls, written summaries before meetings, a combination?

- Status reporting: I would like you to keep me up to date on how you're doing and where you are in relation to the timeline we've established. How would you prefer to keep me up to date?

- Feedback: How do you like to receive feedback? Written, face-to-face, written summary before face-to-face? And how often?

- Autonomy: How much autonomy or independence do you prefer when you are working on a project?

The point is, people really do differ and need their own approaches. Some like their manager to be hands-on. Some learn better when they try things on their own. Some respond best if you give them a few hints and suggestions. Others need to be walked through a project or task step-by-step. To be a good coach, you must tailor your approach to meet individual needs, and if you don't ask, you won't know.

Remember, as a coach you want to help your people become more effective and self-sufficient. You want them to learn to solve their own problems and begin to trust their own instincts and abilities. As a coach, your job is to support them in their development.

Assuming you have a good sense of who your staff members are as individuals, your next task is to make sure you use this information to set them up for success.

Strategy Three: Set People Up for Success

As we mentioned earlier, some managers feel responsible for every outcome and therefore overwhelmed with this sense of responsibility. Coupled with the fear that employees might make mistakes, it is easy to understand why so many managers have a hard time letting go and not being in total control of the work. What's the answer?

When you want to engage your staff in doing challenging work, you need to create the conditions, clarity, and expectations up front that make them likely to perform the tasks successfully.

What do you need to consider? There are loads of great reference books sharing tips on delegation. Exhibit 4.2 gives four tips we hope you will consider the next time you want to let go.

These tips may seem obvious, and perhaps you do consider similar factors when you think through projects and tasks. Why, then, do jobs end up undone and back on your desk? Why do people have difficulty following through and achieving

Exhibit 4.2. Delegation Tips.

1. *Choose worthy projects.* Busywork won't do. Ask yourself if anyone should be doing the job in the first place. If not, eliminate the task.
2. *Match skills and interests.* Choose people who can do the jobs or want to learn how. Try matching people who have certain skills with others on your team who want to learn them.
3. *Consider training.* Think about the training your people need to do a great job. Figure out how they can get this knowledge: from you? from others on the team?
4. *Plan how to monitor and measure progress.* How are you going to check in? Choose simple success indicators that let people know if they are on the right track and what they need to do to make a course correction.

results? Because delegating isn't so easy. Again, different strokes for different folks. Our twist is to ask people to think of all the things they are afraid of, all the things that they feel could go wrong, and together work out a prevention plan.

⚙ Tool: What Could Get in the Way?

Purpose. This tool elicits valuable information from the employee, which helps you anticipate and remove roadblocks to successful completion of the task or project you've delegated to the person.

Method. Ask the employee, "What do you think might get in your way or make this effort difficult for you?"

After asking this open-ended question, dig for specifics by posing possible roadblocks (Exhibit 4.3), hearing the employee's concerns, and addressing them as well as you can at this early point. Typical roadblocks may relate to these issues:

- Unclear goals and guidelines
- Red tape
- Not enough time
- Lack of cooperation from others
- Insufficient access to you for help and support
- All criticism, no praise or appreciation

Exhibit 4.3. Navigating Roadblocks.

If This Is a Concern . . .	. . . Try This:
Unclear goals and guidelines	Take pains to clarify the goals.
	• What does the job or project entail?
	• Why is the job or project important?
	• How does the job fit into the big picture?
	• What do you expect the results to look like?
Red tape	Clarify the employee's latitude to act.
	• No tape: just do it.
	• Pink tape: tell me what you did.
	• Red tape: get permission from me first.
	• Duct tape: forget it.
Not enough time	Negotiate; meet employee half way.
	• Rearrange schedules. Release person from a commitment.
	• Take over a job of theirs.
	• Divide the project into small pieces.
Lack of cooperation from others	Pave the way.
	• Make your team aware of what the person is doing and how it relates to the big picture.
	• Help people feel responsible for each other's success.
	• Help people talk about what they need from each other to accomplish the goal.

Exhibit 4.3. (continued)

If This Is a Concern . . .	. . . Try This:
Insufficient access to you for help and support	Be available.

- Tell person specific ways they can have access to you (e-mail, secretaries, voice mail, and closed doors can all be *barriers!*).
- Ask staff what they think blocks their access to you.

  Announce clear office hours (e.g., three times a week minimum or during a specific hour daily).

  Post times during the week when staff can meet with you.

  Arrange clear and frequent check-in points (whether in writing or face-to-face, depending on what you and your staff prefer).

  Pick a project a week and give feedback to each person working on that project during that week.

  Ask people for feedback. Ask them to list things they view as "on target" or "giving them difficulty," and provide feedback to them about their list.

| All criticism, no positive feedback | Celebrate and praise; talk about what's on target before you point out problems. |

- Write short, encouraging notes ("Keep up the good work!").
- Point out people's accomplishments in public forums.
- Create a "wall of fame" bulletin board in your department.
- Post thank-you letters.
- Celebrate with a "halfway" or midpoint project lunch.

Our core point: you need to set up the task or project and the coaching relationship such that your employees can succeed and you can gain trust in their work. Your up-front investment pays off in results, optimal performance, and a strong relationship with the individuals.

Strategy Four: Create Opportunities for Learning and Course Correction

Of all of the behaviors we've discussed so far, none is as important as how the coach can help people learn and grow from their experience. When your employees have positive experiences, you need to help them reflect on what they learned and understand why they were successful. If they do not meet expectations, you need to help them understand what happened and what would create a different and better outcome. Your challenge is to:

- Recognize opportunities for coaching
- Avoid directing; instead, ask the right questions so people can learn for themselves without feeling disrespected or undermined
- Provide constructive, supportive feedback rather than punishing or causing the employee to feel scolded, judged, or disrespected

Granted, there's a lot to remember. But an effective coaching interaction can go a long way in helping your staff feel good about their accomplishments and learn ways to perform even better. Because this is so important, we suggest that you think through what you want to do and say to bring out the best in people *before* you engage in a coaching session. This allows you to plan the points you know you have to make and the questions you can use to promote the required dialogue. Here is a model for a coaching interaction—a model you can use to plan the interaction and stay on course.

Tool: Coaching Model

Purpose. This tool guides you through coaching interactions with a model that helps you avoid directive behavior.

Method. Use the coaching model below to plan ahead for coaching interactions. Also, take this model with you into a coaching session to remind you of the steps in a constructive, respectful approach.

Model for Coaching Interaction

Process Step	Why This Step Is Important
Describe the issue and why it is important.	People need to see the big picture.
Invite the employee's point of view on both the issue and performance.	People need to feel heard and validated. There may be different sides to the issue.
Invite employee to generate ideas and solutions.	People need to be part of the solution.
Respect, acknowledge, and build on the employee's ideas.	People need you to support their ideas *and* guide and direct them in new ways.
Summarize and agree on a plan.	Both of you need a shared vision to avoid misunderstanding.
Work together to identify responsibilities and time lines; keep maximum responsibility with employee.	People need to be clear on their commitments and responsibilities.
Build employee's confidence and self-esteem all the while.	People need to know you have faith in their abilities.

Practice the coaching model often, and you will become comfortable with the process. Take notes after your coaching sessions and reflect on them, looking for ways to improve. Think about when you felt you were on track and when you felt lost or unsure of what to say. Consider the coaching tips in Exhibit 4.4 as you fine-tune your skills.

As you can see, there is a lot to effective coaching. No wonder telling and directing appear so much easier.

Go, Team!

We know there is lots more to say about coaching, but because the written word is a one-way communication process and good coaching is *two-way*, we can only accomplish so much here. The tools we have shared are basic. The challenge is to deliberately employ them. After all, you, your team, your customers, and your organization have a great deal to gain from your becoming a determined, energetic, frequent, and effective coach who taps into the talents and motivation to learn and stretch that the good people in health care bring with them to work.

Exhibit 4.4. Coaching Tips.

- *Ask questions.* Help staff open up by asking open-ended, not yes-or-no, questions. Talk less and question more.

- *Don't judge.* People shut down if they feel criticized or labeled. Make sure you state your feedback and observations constructively.

- *Listen carefully.* Try to absorb the meaning behind the words. Don't make assumptions. Ask people to explain so you are sure you understand. "Tell me more" is a nonthreatening way to get people to elaborate.

- *Maintain an open mind.* There are usually several ways to achieve a goal. Suspend disbelief, and try to understand the employee's approach if it differs from yours. Give people space to experiment.

- *Show support.* Praise and build on their ideas. "Yes!" and "Good idea!" encourage people to continue the dialogue.

- *Focus on the person.* Talk about yourself and your experiences sparingly. You won't develop others by talking about yourself at length.

- *Avoid comparisons.* Use examples carefully. People don't like to be compared to other people. Watch out for saying "When Mary and her group did this. . . ."

- *Slow down.* People won't open up if they feel rushed. Most people need time to assemble and express their thoughts, feelings, and ideas.

- *Eliminate distractions.* Your employees will not feel valued if you are distracted or doing other things when you are supposed to be talking with them. Don't allow phones, beepers, e-mail alerts, or other people to interrupt this protected time.

- *Less is more.* People can't focus on too many issues at once. Center each discussion on one or two key topics at a time, and build on them in later discussions.

- *Be supportive.* Make sure you are not coming across as intimidating or threatening when you offer suggestions. If you want something done in a certain way, make sure you explain what and why.

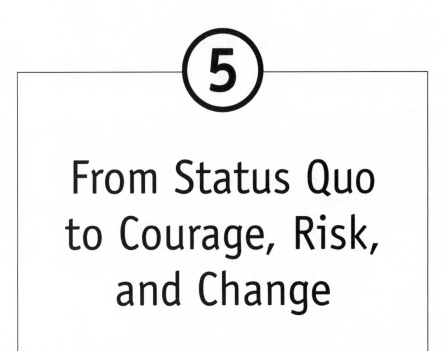

From Status Quo to Courage, Risk, and Change

In today's turbulent environment, you have to be expert in your particular line of business and on top of the changes happening in your marketplace. You also have to advocate for and implement change within your domain of influence and in the domains that intersect with yours. Gone are the days when higher-ups dictate everything you need to do. To be effective, you must step forward and courageously take risks, embrace change, and lead your team members in being optimistic and effective change makers along with you.

A Revealing Look in the Mirror

True or False?	True	False
1. I wait until I have all the facts before making a change or a decision.	____	____
2. I try to maintain a low profile in our organization.	____	____
3. I find myself holding back because of the time and energy it takes to make change happen in our organization or system.	____	____
4. I am uncomfortable when open discussion and disagreement occur within our team.	____	____
5. I find myself focusing more on why things won't work than on what would happen if they did.	____	____
6. I stick my neck out for things that matter to me.	____	____
7. I am usually able to sell my ideas and get people on board with change.	____	____
8. Others view me as a go-getter, someone who makes things happen.	____	____
9. I am sensitive to what people have to go through to embrace change.	____	____
10. I view mistakes as opportunities to learn and grow.	____	____

If you answered false to the first five questions and true to the remaining five, you probably are comfortable with change and may even thrive on it. You are able to make decisions even without all information. You are not afraid to advocate for change, and you mobilize others to embrace it along with you. You are not hesitant to devote time to it, even though this can be consuming. You realize that a work in progress creates inevitable anxiety and risk. You recognize that change is hard for many people, and your sensitivity shows. You also accept that change involves mistakes, which you see in a positive light as opportunity for learning and growth. If this is true for you, consider yourself fortunate, because in today's environment the only constant is change.

It's a New Day

It used to be that a few individuals managed health care organizations. These leaders tended to make the decisions, call the shots, and hold the cards. Managers accepted their authority without question; top-down leadership was the prevailing style. Several senior leaders we have known jokingly call those the good old days, because decisions were easy to make and simple to implement. Most important, the consequence of failure was "Oh, well."

What's changed? Just about everything! Our world is far more complex, our challenges more compelling, the pace of change accelerated, and the environment dynamic. Every day presents new challenges and opportunities. The result is that one leader, or even a few, can't do it all. They don't have the information, skill mix, or time to make things happen without help and support from every other member on the team. More people need to be involved in the process, and more people need to be responsible and accountable for making change happen.

That's not all. Whereas leaders used to feel they could command and control the outcome, today's leaders have to make sure that people are on board, that they are engaged in the process, that they understand what they need to do to be successful, and that they have the support required to do it. Hard? Absolutely!

Take a Look

Let's look at the shift from status quo to courage, risk, and change in some real situations.

Ken

Ken identifies a need to change his service's scheduling system to shorten the patient waiting time. He knows that he'd better involve certain key physicians whose personal schedules would be affected.

Recognizing this need, some status quo–oriented managers would simply do nothing, thinking *Who needs this grief?* Realizing that certain powerful individuals might go around and above them to preserve their preferred schedules, that these same individuals would probably cause a scene and complain to others, or worse that they would sabotage the new process, such managers might find it hard to psych themselves up to make waves.

But Ken, a change-adept leader, knows that customer satisfaction is the key, and that doing nothing to relieve patient waiting time is unacceptable. He also knows that he must bring the physicians on board carefully. He does his homework, collects the facts, cultivates possible physician allies, and makes the case from a position of strength. Also, understanding that there are many ways to skin a cat, Ken is open to alternative approaches, as long as they do not compromise the goal of reducing wait time.

Kelly

Kelly's boss has asked her to implement a change in her area. Although she agrees with the change philosophically, she knows that it will create difficulties for her staff, particularly at this time.

In this situation, some managers might feel oppressed, moving forward with the change reluctantly and letting the administration be the fall guys. They would likely present the change as something "they are making us do." They would begrudgingly proceed to do it.

As a change leader, Kelly knows that the change is right but the timing wrong. Either she makes a case for changing or modifying the schedule or, after thinking about it further, she concludes that there may never be a better time. Rather than postponing the inevitable, she decides to move forward with the change. She then maps out a long-range implementation plan that enables her team to tackle the project one step at a time. She doesn't let her team off the hook, but she finds a healthy way to surface and address their fears and resistance.

Kelly is able to see a variety of alternatives. When her staff realizes that she is listening to their concerns and taking a stand for what needs to be done, they respect her and feel respected by her. Kelly demonstrates both courage and sensitivity to her team's reality.

Kim

Kim has developed what she believes is a better way to perform one of her department's key functions. She has mapped out a trial run and involved her staff in its implementation. But lo and behold, the new way creates more problems than it solves.

Duck and cover, run and hide would be the M.O. of the risk-averse manager. Of course, it doesn't feel good to fail, but these leaders wear their failures like a shield, protecting themselves from future opportunity to learn and make improvements. Another response from managers uncomfortable with change might be to point the finger; if something goes wrong, it must be someone else's fault. Usually, the someone else is another department or "administration." Regardless, these managers are trying to escape blame by blaming others, so they can feel better about what they would otherwise perceive as their own failure.

But Kim, a change-adept manager, can reframe failure. She learns from the experience of implementing the change and makes sure that her team shares the learning. Early on, she puts in place systems to let her know how they are doing, so she and her team can make course corrections, tweaking their plans as they go along to turn what might otherwise be an unsuccessful outcome into an effective change. Even in the face of disappointing results, she doesn't abandon the effort. She says, "Given what we're seeing, how can we fine-tune our approach to make it work?"

Some managers might see to it that trial runs and pilot programs actually do fail, knowing that if the project is abandoned, they won't have to change the way they do things enduringly. But Kim sees a trial run as an enlightening first step along an inevitable journey to important improvement.

Ken, Kelly, and Kim have the guts to lead change with their teams. They stick their necks out. They are able to chart new frontiers despite the risks and uncertainties involved.

What Worries You?

Are you uncomfortable making waves? Making waves and rocking the boat can be uncomfortable. You might draw attention to you or your cause, and perhaps you don't like to be the center of attention or controversy. You might feel most at ease by going along with and supporting the party line.

Do you find yourself anxious in the face of ongoing uncertainty? If you don't like surprises, you might find the uncertainty associated with making change disconcerting or anxiety-provoking. Or you may find it hard to deal with other people's anxiety if you are feeling unsure or insecure yourself.

Are you a perfectionist? In the process of change, things can and will go wrong. If you have a need to be perfect, if you are uncomfortable making mistakes, you might prefer to avoid risk—especially one that could become public. How are you with risk?

Does your need for approval make it hard for you to handle people's negative feelings? Change breeds controversy. People accept change at different rates and in their own ways. You may find it difficult dealing with the personal issues and agendas that arise as people go through the stages of accepting change. If you have a big need to be liked, this might be unsettling for you.

Are you uncomfortable with conflict? Because some people never get on board with the change, you must prepare yourself to deal with many kinds of resistance. This can be particularly difficult if the people whose support you require are peers and bosses. If you are uncomfortable with conflict, this might also deter you from embracing the role of change leader.

Are you afraid you won't be up to the task involved? Leading change may require you to leave your own comfort zone. You might fear getting in over your head. Needing new skills, you may fear that either you don't have what it takes or you don't have the time and resources to get the support to pull off the change.

Finally, are you concerned about being overly accountable? If *you* initiate the change, if *you* take the lead, you can't point the finger at anyone else should things not turn out well. It can be lonely on top of Change Mountain, and this stops lots of managers from making the climb.

What Do You Stand to Gain?

Putting it bluntly, we really are living in a change-or-die environment. You have to change to keep up. You also need to make sure that your people are keeping up. Despite the downside of becoming a change leader, you have a lot to gain (starting with survival, but there are many other benefits as well).

- *You will develop "change muscles."* When you are a change leader, you don't process disappointing results as failure. You view yourself as an experimenter who is trying new things, fine-tuning, and making course corrections, learning along the way. If change leadership is not your normal mode, you might feel some angst as you experience the first few disappointing outcomes, but after weathering a few such storms you realize you are surviving and so you get better at both accepting and leading change. With experience, spearheading change becomes much easier, less frightening, and even exciting.

- *When you lead change, you grow.* You have an opportunity to stretch and expand your skills and experience. Many people find this energizing, since boredom can lead to personal and organizational burnout.

- *Change means opportunity.* When you shake things up, you get an opportunity to tackle sticky issues, even if it means rattling people who probably should have been disturbed a long time ago. Some of us relish this as an opportunity, once and for all, to make a positive difference.

- *You'll earn people's admiration.* Because all managers feel the pressure to lead changes, when you make the shift to change leader others view you with respect. You show them that you embrace change and continue on energetically, and this eases their way.
- *You'll make yourself more marketable.* More often than not, an organization's honchos want to hire individuals who are not afraid of controversy, who can make change happen, and who can lead others into a new frontier that better serves the mission and goals—and that, deviating from the way things have always been, adds value and gains distinction for the organization.

What Can You Do? How Can You Do It?

We realize that change leadership is complicated and not easy. We recommend here four strategies to help you embrace change and become a leader of others in the process (Exhibit 5.1).

Exhibit 5.1. Your Courage, Risk, and Change Toolkit.

Strategy one: Think like a change leader, addressing your own fears and commitment.

Strategy two: Understand and reduce the risks involved.

Strategy three: Sell the change to your team.

Strategy four: Make the change happen by planning, implementing, and learning from the journey.

The first strategy helps you think like a change leader. After all, you don't want to be your own worst enemy.

Because change brings with it inherent uncertainty and leadership of it entails certain risks, you have to prepare yourself to manage these risks. Otherwise, you will back away from the challenges of change. The second strategy helps you manage the risks involved.

As change leader, you will frequently be in a position to want to, or have to, gain your team's commitment to change that they are being asked to make or change that affects them. Our third strategy helps you become an effective salesperson for change with your own team and colleagues.

Our fourth strategy helps you navigate the change process, so that you get optimal results and also learn from the process. It equips you with tools you can use to plan, implement, evaluate, and learn from changes you're spearheading.

Strategy One: Think Like a Change Leader

A large part of being an effective change agent involves getting others on board, presenting a winning case for change, and doing so in a way that invites dialogue and engagement. The situations Herb, Kelly, and Kim faced earlier involved controversy, whether it was the physicians who didn't want a new schedule to disrupt their routine, or employees who were afraid of the unknown, or bosses who believed that there is only one way. In each case, the manager needed to personally embrace the change, prepare to sell it, be able to listen with an open mind, and handle resistance in a constructive and balanced fashion.

This is tough unless you think like a change leader: "I can make this happen," or "I can handle the challenges," and even "This is something I want to do." If you yourself have not come to terms with the change or if you feel insecure with yourself and your role, you will have a hard time getting others to follow. That's why we start by sharing several tools you can use to adopt the mind-set of a change leader and ready yourself for the change journey.

✪ Tool: I Have What It Takes!

Purpose. This tool helps you identify previous successes and the internal strengths you have that contributed to them, so that you will be able, in the face of change, to think *I have what it takes.*

Method. Go to a quiet, uncluttered place and set everything else aside. Make sure you have turned off phones and beepers for a short time, so you won't be distracted.

Close your eyes, relax, and take a few deep breaths. Listen to the sound of your breathing as you inhale and exhale. Concentrating on your breathing, think about a time that you made a change effectively. This change could be personal or professional, but the change had a significant effect on you.

Think about this change and reflect on these questions:

- What was the change?
- Why was this change important to you?

- What were your initial thoughts about this change?
- What helped you make this change?
- What were the barriers and obstacles that you had to overcome?
- What were the outcomes, and what did you learn about yourself?

It is important that you begin to understand that you had the power to make a successful change, and you still have that power. What is it? What are the things in you that have helped you embrace change in the past? What resources do you bring to the challenge of making other changes?

This exploration is important as the thoughts you have about yourself and others, the project and the situation, influence what you are willing and not willing to do. If you see yourself as powerful and capable, you are likely to stick your neck out and take the risks needed when charting a new course. If you see yourself as weak or insecure, you may tend to play it safe. This next tool helps you continue examining your inner world as it relates to risk and change.

Tool: My Inner Talk

Purpose. This tool guides you in identifying your thoughts and feelings related to a change you want to make and their impact on the likelihood that you'll move ahead.

Method. Think about a change you want to make. Make sure you have a strong personal connection to this change. It should not be something that others want for you, but something that you want personally or professionally.

Jot down your thoughts about your ability to be successful in making this change, such as:

- I've done this before.
- This will be easy for me to do.
- I know how to do this.
- Others have done this, and they've survived.
- I have resources to help me.

- I'll learn from this.
- I know this is important for me.

Now, jot down any thoughts you have that might make this change difficult for you, such as:

- I have other things on my plate.
- I'm not sure if I can pull this off.
- This will be harder than I think.
- I'll need a great deal of support.
- I don't know how to do this.
- I could get in trouble.
- I could look bad.
- I could lose a great deal.
- I will be alone.

Look over both lists. Which thoughts are your dominant ones? Are they the thoughts that help you move on with the change, or the ones that hold you back?

How do you feel about yourself when you think the thoughts on the positive list? How about the ones on the negative list?

For any inhibiting thoughts, consider where they might have come from. Now hold a one-person debate in an effort to talk yourself out of thinking this way.

Finally, write down, read, and reread three thoughts that you want to hold in awareness more often because you believe they support you as a change leader.

Without being aware of it, you are influenced by the thoughts and feelings you have about yourself, others, and the situation. By getting a grip on them, you can choose what to think, and think thoughts that help you in your change leadership role. But wait! There's more to understand about your inner world. This next tool helps you put the entire process in perspective by looking at what you have to lose.

⚒ Tool: What Have I Got to Lose?

Purpose. This tool helps you pinpoint your fears and put them into perspective, so that they don't prevent you from taking risks or moving forward.

Method. Think about a risky change you want to make, or a person you need to confront. Think about these words, and circle the ones you feel or fear might be on the line if you take the risk. Think *worst-case* possibility. What might you risk?

- Job security
- Boss's approval
- Career options
- Information
- Income
- Image in the group
- Control
- Authority
- Peer support
- Respect of others
- Friendships
- Affection of others
- Team spirit
- Staff commitment

Look over your list and ask yourself, How realistic are these possibilities? Which ones are really likely to happen? Which ones would be a problem for you or your group if they did happen? Why do you think this?

Consider whether there is any way you could be mistaken about these fears. Is there any way that you could be exaggerating? Also, if these fears come true, do you have a way of handling the consequences?

Consider how these fears may be holding you back or keeping you from doing what you need to do. Consider that your fears are not the same as reality. They are *fears*!

We have found great comfort in doing this worst-case-scenario thinking. In most instances, the worst case you can think of is either highly improbable or, if it were to happen, might not be nearly as catastrophic as you feel, because you have an effective way you can handle it. A good friend of ours once confided that she was afraid of losing her job if she confronted her boss and spoke out for what she felt was right. This leader had been holding back for a long time and been miserable in the process. Her relationship with her boss was not one of mutual respect. Because she was not appreciated for her gifts, she often talked about leaving. Only fear of the unknown kept her in this stuck place.

The worst case for her was not that she could lose her job; the worst case for her was *not* losing her job. Keeping her job was the worst thing that could happen to her. This is certainly not easy for people to see, but it's often a reality that they come to acknowledge. Many people who lose their jobs end up considering it a blessing in disguise. They say, had they known what they now know, they would have left the uncomfortable situation much sooner.

If you look back at times in your life when you feared catastrophic consequences of something you wanted to do, but you proceeded to do it anyway, you will probably agree that the extent of your fears proved to be unwarranted and that you indeed had the internal resources to handle adverse consequences better than you thought. Fortunately, you'll find that to be true of your fears about change leadership.

Strategy Two: Understand and Reduce the Risks Involved

Understanding your fears and what holds you back are important first steps. Your next step is to consider the risks involved for you and your team and figure out how you can minimize them, so they are not debilitating.

We love this next tool. It helps you get the cards on the table and directly manage any resistance to change that you encounter among your team or colleagues rather than being blocked or intimidated by it. This is a powerful risk-reduction technique, since the greatest risks are often sabotage or inertia among the very people whom you want to work with you to make the change happen.

⚒ Tool: How Can We Mess This Up?

Purpose. This tool helps you address the resistance to change you and your team members express. It helps engage the skeptics on your team to express their concerns directly to you, instead of to each other in the parking lot. With this tool, your team sees that there are ways to prevent many of the negative outcomes they expect. The tool yields valuable information that enables you to strengthen your original plan.

Method. Focusing your team on a change that is or will be occurring, ask the members to don their skeptic hats and brainstorm all the ways that they (or anyone) could prevent this change from being a success. List their responses on a flipchart or wallboard.

Ask team members to rate the responses on these criteria:

- Which ones are likely to occur?
- Which ones would have the most negative effect if they did occur?
- Pick the top winners and do some prevention planning.
- If this did occur, how could we minimize the effect?
- How could we prevent this from happening altogether?

This tool helps you replace why-we-can't energy with how-we-can energy, making it much more likely that you will pull off the change to everyone's satisfaction. The next tool reduces risk differently: by surrounding you with support, so that you are not alone in dealing with whatever the trials and tribulations of the change process happen to be.

Consider Ralph. He is a manager Gail worked with who was in the process of integrating two radiology groups. He had been avoiding working with his team to redesign roles and responsibilities, even though his boss was pressing him to offer new services without adding personnel. Ralph knew he couldn't just roll over and say yes. His people were already complaining about being overworked and stressed. Needing to be liked by everyone, he felt uncomfortable asking his staff to do more. He was afraid he would alienate them and lose their cooperation. He was not atypical. He was afraid of becoming isolated and alone.

The next tool is an exercise that helps you identify resources available to support you as you lead change, so that you will not feel alone. Most managers feel isolated and alone, not because they are but because they don't think to engage the resources around them, be they staff, peers, or leaders.

✪ Tool: Where's the Support?

Purpose. This tool helps you think about the resources and supports you can tap to help you lead change. It helps you think about how to use the talents and resources you have available.

Method. Turn off your phone, beeper, and other distractions. Take a few moments to relax. Close your eyes and concentrate on your breathing. Take a few deep breaths and listen to the sounds you make as you inhale and exhale.

Think about the people you are comfortable with at work. These are individuals whom you can talk to, whose ideas and opinions you respect. Picture these people and what you value about each one of them.

Now picture other people in your system, those you may see everyday but do not talk to regularly. Think about all of the talent and skills these people have, the resources they bring with them, and the knowledge and understanding they have that you don't even know about.

Next, envision people you have met or talked to at seminars, workshops, and conferences. Think about the talent and skills that they have, their interests and knowledge, and the resources they bring with them also.

Think about the people you know outside of work—your family and friends. Picture these people, and think about the skills and interests they have and the knowledge and resources they offer.

Now, take out a piece of paper and jot down some of the people whose knowledge and skills you *do* use and ways that you tap into this resource. Think also about the people in your life or your network whose interests and knowledge and skills you *could* use, if you made the connections.

Finally, think about the unbelievable amount of talent that actually lies within your reach:

- What would you like to do with this talent?
- How could you access it?
- What holds you back?
- How could you get over that?

Most people find it easy to generate a wide network once they get started, but they limit this network in their daily lives. In truth, you are surrounded by a wealth of resources. Both of us authors see overworked and overstressed managers every day. At the same time, there is a wealth of underused talent that we could tap into if we were willing and could figure out how to do so. In the earlier example, Ralph was not alone. He had resources that he hadn't considered in his own team, and his organization helped him connect to other leaders by creating a management support system. As a result, he ended up with buddies who helped him realistically evaluate his options and figure out ways to move forward with his staff and with his boss.

Strategy Three: Sell the Change to Your Team

Once Ralph began to understand what he and his team had to gain by changing, his next step was to involve them in the change process. He realized he couldn't make anything happen without their commitment and support. To do this effectively, he had to present the change in a way that they would understand and embrace. For most managers, selling a change is difficult and requires a lot of thoughtful planning. Here's a tool to help you think through the process, organizing your thoughts so you can present a winning case.

⚒ Tool: Making Your Case for Change

Purpose. This tool helps you do the homework and prethinking necessary to create your pitch for change, and make the pitch successfully with your team.

Method. Here's the homework that helps you prepare a great pitch for change:

- *What is the change?* Describe the change or outcome you want in one or two sentences (for instance, change a policy, consolidate a particular service line).

- *Why is this change important?* Describe what led up to this change and why it is compelling.

- *What are the costs and benefits?* What are the benefits of this change, for individuals? for the organization? What is the downside of this change? What makes this change difficult?

- *Whose support do you need?* Why should these individuals or groups support this effort? Why would they resist? What concerns could they have?

- *What else is in the way?* What obstacles might you face? What can you do to eliminate them?

- *How should you begin?* Who do you need to sell this to first? What are the key concepts you need to present in the initial meeting? What are the issues you need to get on the table? What are some questions you need to ask or strategies you need to use to make sure this initial meeting is a success?

Sound like a lot of work? Yes, but you need to do your homework to make a great case for change. You have to gather the right facts and anticipate and prepare to address the information needs and concerns among your team to win their support. Once you gather these facts and think through your pitch, we encourage you to try it out on a coworker or friend who can give you feedback and help you fine-tune it. This minimizes your risk and helps you prepare even better. It also helps you practice handling resistance, so you won't be blindsided in the real experience.

Strategy Four: Make the Change Happen by Planning, Implementing, and Learning from the Journey

No matter how much prework you do or how much input you get, no change happens perfectly. We've never seen a change that didn't need to be modified, tweaked, and simplified to work with the current reality. Your role is to be open to the possibilities, and to have feedback and success indicators in place to let people know in real time how the change is going. This is important because the planning phase focuses on concepts and strategy. During planning, people do not need to do anything new or different. All of that changes when you actually install a new process or change.

During the planning phase, people share their resistance by telling you, "This won't work." When you install a change and people experience the inevitable mishaps and difficulties, the resisters often come back this time, saying, "It's not working." You must prepare for this and help your team share their feelings, identify and tackle emerging snags, and experience and savor easy wins. This is a critical part of the change process, but not easy to handle. Many leaders find themselves buckling under the pressure and giving up, thinking, *OK, I tried, it didn't work; I guess it's time to move on.*

Successful leaders realize that resistance is a natural part of the process. They also realize that it is up to them to help their team through the awkward and uncomfortable period of getting used to a new way of doing things. But most of all, successful change agents understand that giving up is denying them and their group an opportunity to learn and grow.

A successful way to address the kind of resistance that is typical of the implementation phase is to strategically implement changes one step at a time. People do need to understand the big picture and direction of the change, but it's easier to swallow the elephant in small bites.

In Ralph's case, there were many changes that had to occur to support the integration process. The most important was to encourage staff to accept changes in leadership and to understand where they fit in. They also needed to create a clear picture of the future, complete with team goals and objectives. And although there were many systems and processes that were to be changed, Ralph had to help his group create a plan and timeline that would push the group but not overwhelm them. The challenge for him was keeping the group on track and not letting the daily routine get in the way. It is one thing to plan the changes, but leaders often back down when staff says, "We're too busy" or "Let's try this during down time."

The next set of tools helped Ralph and can help you keep your team on track.

⚒ Tool: Where Are We Going, and How Will We Get There?

Purpose. This tool helps your team map out a long-range plan for change.

Method. Describe the overall changes that the team needs to make in a few short sentences.

- Describe the end result of these changes. What will the change look like when it is successful? Give yourself a maximum time this change will take and use that time to draw a complete picture ("In two years, here's where we'll be").

- Describe what you think you will have achieved in half that amount of time ("In one year, here is what we will have achieved"). Describe again what you think you will have achieved in half of *that* time.

- Continue, until you are talking about what things must be accomplished in the first few weeks of the change.

This type of planning helps your team see those immediate things they can do to lead up to the overall change. They can see the building blocks of the change, one block at a time. It also helps your team see how they can achieve early victories. Because the cynics will try to pull the rug out from under the team, saying "It's not working," it's important for you to put in place success indicators or tracking devices that give you feedback along the way about how you're doing. These enable you to stay rational and open-minded despite what the cynics might be telling you.

The physicians in Ralph's service were concerned about turnover on the team and losing business during the transition. Ralph realized that both of these concerns would be easy to monitor. He designed a simple survey to take the pulse of the team weekly, in terms of their issues and concerns. Also, the team designed a quick customer comment card for patients to fill out as they were leaving the clinic. The questions he asked the group are listed in Exhibit 5.2.

Exhibit 5.2. Customer Comment Card.

Rate the following issues on a scale of 1 to 5	–				+
How comfortable do you feel with your new role?	1	2	3	4	5
How easy is it for you to do your job?	1	2	3	4	5
How do you feel about the communication in the team?	1	2	3	4	5
How comfortable are you with your new partners?	1	2	3	4	5

Like Ralph, you can use the tool "How Can We Mess This Up?" to unearth your team's worst-case fears. Then, focusing on these fears, do prevention planning and create monitoring devices to measure progress and reassure your team that they and the change implementation process are moving in the right direction.

Ralph also held daily five-minute check-in meetings with his group for the first few weeks. Here, the group talked about things that seemed to be working and one thing the group could do to make that day more successful.

Using these tools, Ralph was surprised by his results. His team was much more comfortable with the changes than he had imagined. He attributed this to the chemistry of the group. But we know that it worked out well because he remained focused on his goals and persisted even in the face of cynicism and resistance. He stayed in people's faces, updated the group in every meeting, charted progress, and didn't back off from the setbacks and failures. Better yet, he helped his team grow by turning these trials into a learning experience.

Helping your team turn trials into a learning experience, helping your team process what's happening and savor progress—these are critical. Here is one of our favorite techniques. You can use this tool at any time, but it's a wonderful way for your team to think back on the last six months or year if they have been through a major change initiative.

✖ Tool: Reflections on Our Journey

Purpose. This tool helps your team talk through the changes that have taken place, to help appreciate (and bury) the past and establish common ground for the future.

Method. Ask your team (in small groups) to think about changes they have been through in, say, the last six to twelve months. Use the questions below to guide their discussion.

Question Guide

1. How did we begin our journey?

2. What happened in the early stages of the journey? What happened to individuals?
   to the team?

3. What challenges and obstacles have we faced?

4. What have we accomplished?

5. What did we have to change or let go of to continue on our journey?

6. What did we learn from our experience? Where are we now? Where will our journey
   continue to take us?

Some of your people may feel uncomfortable going through an exercise like this, thinking it is too touchy-feely. Don't back down. It is a healthy ritual for your group to take time out, acknowledge the challenges they've tackled, celebrate their accomplishments, and connect to one another around their shared future.

Taking Risks and Managing Change with Courage

With so much change going on in, between, and around health care organizations, the only sign on your organization's door that remains accurate over time is the one that reads "Subject to Change Without Notice." Shifting from comfort with the status quo to risk taking and managing tumultuous change takes dedication on your part—dedication to your goals and your team. Paradoxically, it takes planning and stick-to-itiveness combined with flexibility and agility to change course. It takes determination and guts. It takes tolerating ambiguity. It takes savvy in the face of inevitable resistance. It takes humility. It takes an un-self-conscious commitment to learning and making course corrections along the way. In short, it challenges leaders. It requires leadership. It is an opportunity to show leadership strength.

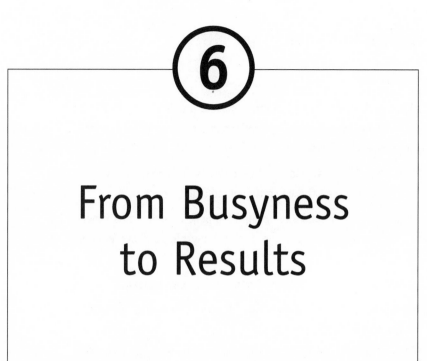

From Busyness to Results

Because of the demands on us in today's health care environment, the financial constraints that limit our access to resources, and the speed with which our society and competitors act, busyness doesn't cut it anymore. These days, it's results that count: benefits for customers and your organization that you produce in a timely fashion and at a high standard.

A Revealing Look in the Mirror

True or False?	True	False
1. I do my homework so well before I make a proposal that by the time I make my case, I'm confident that the proposal is worthwhile.	____	____
2. When I can't meet a deadline, I renegotiate it instead of saying nothing and hoping the person involved won't notice.	____	____
3. When I'm trying to make something happen, I commit to a time line so that I stay focused and don't let anything and everything take priority.	____	____
4. I aggressively solve problems; I don't just identify them.	____	____
5. When I'm going to run a meeting, I prepare thoroughly so that every minute is well spent.	____	____
6. If I were to list my actual accomplishments for the past year, it would be a short list, because most things are a work in progress.	____	____
7. I find it hard to make process improvements quickly, because so many people need to be involved.	____	____
8. I find it difficult not to respond to the daily crisis and stay focused on my priorities.	____	____
9. I have a hard time holding other people to their commitments.	____	____
10. I don't leave a meeting without clear next steps.	____	____

If you answered true to the first five statements and false to the last five, you seem to function as a results-oriented manager. You are not only inclined to work hard and expend considerable effort as busyness-oriented managers do, but you also persist and push for results and have accomplishment to show for it.

As a results-oriented manager, you have a clear vision of results, and you judge your value to the organization by these outcomes, not by how hard you work. You are concerned about turnaround time for a decision or project, and you get impatient when it drags on and on. You are likely to be decisive, clear in your expectations, and open to finding the best people to help you. You tend to hold yourself accountable by tracking your results and keeping yourself on schedule.

You are clear about commitments, and when you can't keep them, you renegotiate. You make meetings matter, preparing for them well so that the group has a better chance of reaching a conclusion or decision. When you see a problem, you go after it. When you initiate or participate in problem solving or process improvement, you maintain focus on the goal until there is a solution or an experiment to try. You are intolerant of seemingly endless meetings and processes.

In contrast, if you are busyness-oriented, you no doubt work hard but not necessarily with efficiency or purpose. You are prone to seeing your job in quantitative terms, as hours in the day, number of problems to solve, items on a to-do list, the height of the stack in your in-basket, the number of e-mail messages and meetings. You make excuses for not finishing a task or meeting a commitment. You slow down in the face of obstacles instead of forging ahead. You allow yourself to be distracted from what you say are your priorities. Sometimes you strive to complete a task quickly to get it over with or off your to-do list, regardless of the extent to which it fulfills a purpose.

It's a New Day

Does this scenario look familiar? A group of managers are on a standing committee. They schedule their monthly meetings into their calendars and plan other things around them. At each meeting, they grab a cup of coffee, sink into a chair, and begin by asking, "So, where were we?" They rehash where they left off, share a few off-the-cuff reports, and throw some ideas around, until someone remarks that their time is nearly up and that they should decide what happens next. They often conclude by agreeing to continue the discussion at the next meeting.

What's remarkable about this scenario? No results. Nada. Nothing. Yet these people believe they are working! If they reflect on it, they might admit that every meeting is a welcome break from their hectic work, even if it is unproductive. The point is, keeping busy and even running ragged are not the same as adding value.

This kind of dynamic characterizes many committees, improvement teams, task forces, and councils month after month and year after year, even when these groups accomplish very little. In the old days, showing up was enough, because there was so much less pressure to make things happen rapidly. But no more. Today, it's results that count.

Take a Look

Here are four managers in four situations. Take a look at how they handle the situation depending on whether they act as someone busyness-oriented or results-oriented.

Susan

Susan runs an outpatient surgery center in a hotly competitive health care market-place. Like every department in the medical center of which the surgicenter is a part, Susan's has a quality improvement team that sets and monitors quality stan-dards and pursues improvement projects.

As a busyness-oriented manager, Susan makes sure the quality team meets reg-ularly and documents its goals, data, and decisions. She keeps the pressure on the team leader to engage the team in defining improvement opportunities and pur-suing them methodically, even if people are swamped and therefore spread the work of the project across many months. Susan thinks, *Slow and steady progress wins the race,* and always has good work-in-progress to show the surveyors from the Joint Commission for the Accreditation of Healthcare Organizations during their visit every three years.

If Susan were results-oriented, not busyness oriented, she would also attend to quality, but differently. To compete effectively in the environment in which this sur-gicenter operates, she is keenly aware that she must spearhead *rapid* improvement that creates visible positive effects for patients and other customers. She is less con-cerned about the validity and reliability of data and more concerned that the team is triggering active experimentation, with pilots and trial runs and frequent hud-dles regarding progress. She recognizes that speed is critical to competitive success.

Bob

Bob goes to his boss, Milt, and says he needs a laptop to make someone in his office more efficient. Milt says he'll consider it if Bob brings him data justifying the increase in efficiency. Bob goes back to his department, develops the analysis, and presents it to Milt at his next meeting. Milt says, "Very interesting, but isn't there another computer in the department that he could use, so we wouldn't have to spend money on this?" While Bob answers, Milt isn't satisfied and asks him to bring to their next meeting a list of who has computers and how they use them, as well as an analysis of downtime on these computers. Bob sighs at the thought of all that work for what appears to be a no-brainer, but he agrees to do it because he wants approval on the computer. When he returns with the answer, Milt still isn't satisfied and asks Bob to find out how departments in other hospitals perform this same function. Bob says he'll make some calls to contacts and get back to him.

Meanwhile, Bob is disgusted. He confides in someone, "This is a no-brainer. It's not that expensive. And I have to go through all these hoops to get an answer. For-get it. We'll be inefficient. I give up." He proceeds to manage his function knowing it is sorely inefficient. He also stands to lose a good employee by not giving her the tools she needs to do her job.

Some people would say Milt is being ridiculous, and maybe so. But focus on Bob's approach instead of Milt's. He probably should know by now that Milt doesn't make decisions until he feels he has *all* the information. If Bob were a results-oriented manager, he would do more homework up front, bringing Milt a comprehensive case for the computer early on and speeding up the boss's approval process. By not doing this, Bob becomes demoralized, giving up after spending a load of time on gathering information for Milt—all to no avail.

Paula

Paula feels ambitious and takes on hard problems that affect her team's ability to do its job. But her team members think nothing ever changes. They hear Paula say repeatedly, "I'm working on it. It takes time." As time wears on and Paula doesn't make any changes related to the hard problems, her staff members feel increasingly helpless. Paula is a great person and seems to care, but she does not make things happen for her staff, and they know this. Her day is filled with immediate requests from her boss, checking e-mail, and responding to phone messages. Before she knows it, her day is over, and she hasn't spent any time on her priority projects.

If Paula were results-oriented, she would persist and bring things to fruition for her staff, and they would respect and appreciate her for it. She would not make excuses. She would recognize that her team relies on her to advocate for the conditions, processes, and tools they need to do their jobs well. She would put their needs on a fast track, avoid other distraction, and proceed to test improvements and approaches responsive to their needs.

Dave

Dave's department is high on the priority list for the forthcoming accreditation visit by JCAHO. Although he knew to expect this site visit for more than a year, he was so busy with pressing things that he did nothing to prepare. Now, the JCAHO is coming and he is in a panic. In a crisis mode, he badgers his staff to stay late, work harder, and make everything ready—on an impossible timeline.

Busyness-oriented, Dave has devoted his time and energy to other things all year and now has no choice but to consider the Joint Commission visit a crisis. He proceeds to order people around in a wild frenzy to pass inspection, letting his other priorities go by the wayside entirely.

A results-oriented manager would have foreseen and planned for the Joint Commission visit. He would not have waited for them to be knocking at the door. He would have created a plan over many months—a plan that would have made it possible to continue business as usual by the time the Joint Commission arrived. He would have created his own deadlines and integrated them with his team's other priorities.

What Worries You?

Getting results seems to be a critical challenge in most organizations. Where are managers stuck?

Is the norm in your organization to be busy, overworked, and swamped, causing people with a results orientation to be shunned or quietly resented? Some managers don't push for results for fear that they will be resented by those who don't demand results at all.

Do you like the excuse of being swamped? Some people want an easy excuse to use when others expect something of them. If you're swamped, you can say no to other people's requests. Busyness keeps people at a distance, afraid to ask anything of you.

Do you avoid confrontation? To bring about results, you might have to behave in a way that irritates or pushes others to perform or produce. If you don't push, you can remain Mr. or Ms. Nice Guy. Knowing that you have to assert yourself sometimes to get others to meet their commitments, you may back away from results because you don't want to confront other people who are letting you down.

Do you fear that others will judge your results once you finally deliver them? Some people feel insecure about their ability to produce results.

Do you enjoy checking lots of things off your to-do list? Some people focus on the little things, the less important things, to experience "closure" on certain tasks, all the while producing no results *important* to the organization.

Are you afraid you'll run out of things to do if you finish the main items on your plate? Some people think *As long as I'm still working on something, I'll continue to be needed.* They make it their business to stay busy, busy, busy.

Are you afraid that the next task will be even harder? Some managers, were they to be challenged, might protest, "If I don't complete my priority projects, then I don't have to stretch or challenge myself to do the next thing, which might be harder or even frightening."

Does being frantically busy make you feel indispensable? Perhaps seeing your endless to-do list makes you feel important and needed.

The hitch is that unless you visibly help your organization achieve results, your value to the organization is in jeopardy. Executives want tangible outcomes that advance the organization's goals. Customers want services to be delivered with quality, efficiency, and timeliness, without excuses. The focus on results is really about accountability.

What Do You Stand to Gain?

The choice is yours. Think about these benefits of a results orientation, and hopefully you will be convinced.

- *You make things happen.* When you hold yourself accountable and produce results, you have accomplishments you can point to—a track record—and a reason for pride.

- *People rely on you and respect you.* Others in the organization know they can rely on you to make things happen, to complete things, to produce.

- *You experience the joy of closure.* Your to-do list actually gets shorter! You reduce the anxiety that busyness-oriented managers feel as they look at the hard and important things on their to-do lists day after day without seeing any of them drop off the list.

- *You see change and improvement.* You see your impact. All of this earns you the respect of others and makes you more promotable and marketable.

- *Your staff members learn from you and appreciate your effectiveness.* You no doubt want your own staff to be effective. When you are, you set the pace for them to follow. You'll see more productivity from your team when they see more of it from you.

- *You can maintain balance and perspective.* When you're frantically busy, you no doubt feel pushed and pulled, out of control, reactive and tired. When you produce results, you can take a break, step back, and appreciate what you've done.

What Can You Do? How Can You Do It?

We hope you're convinced that busyness is overrated and that you can benefit by becoming an even more results-oriented manager. If so, here are six strategies to help you make the transition (Exhibit 6.1).

Exhibit 6.1. Your Results Orientation Toolkit.

Strategy one: Think results!

Strategy two: Prepare for results.

Strategy three: Focus and fend off interruptions.

Strategy four: Speed up to produce results.

Strategy five: Go after results in meetings.

Strategy six: Finish.

The first strategy helps you embrace beliefs about yourself and your work that support a results orientation. You examine your thoughts and replace any that favor busyness in lieu of results.

The second strategy acquaints you with tools for envisioning your goals and planning whenever getting results appears scary or difficult.

The third strategy includes some of our favorite ways to keep your focus and to fend off the multitude of interruptions that stand between you and results.

The fourth strategy addresses speed, offering you tools for making rapid cycle changes and improvements.

Since we don't dare ignore the importance of meetings in achieving results, with the fifth strategy we show you tools for making meetings productive or worth their weight in results.

Finally, with strategy number six, we harangue you on the importance of finishing; a lot of great work never sees the light of day because managers don't do the last steps that bring it to closure.

So, there's lots of exercise coming up for you if you want to build your result-getting muscles.

Strategy One: Think Results

The first strategy for mobilizing you toward results, results, results may involve an adjustment in your thinking. Do you think thoughts or hold beliefs that stop or deter you from going after results with a vengeance? This next tool helps you pinpoint any such thoughts and replace them with ones that move you in a results-oriented direction.

⚒ Tool: What Thoughts or Beliefs Trip You Up?

Purpose. This tool helps you consider the psychological obstacles that stand between you and getting results.

Method. In the middle column of the lists below, check the statements that reflect thoughts you have about yourself.

What Thoughts Trip You Up?

Thought	Yes, I Think This!	I Would Be Better Off If I Thought This Instead
The challenges I face are *hard*. I don't know *how* to get the results I want, and I hesitate to admit it.		I can get help without losing people's respect. I'll lose respect if I *don't* get this done.
It's a rare project that I can accomplish without the cooperation of others. To get results, I have to push other people to do their part, and I don't like to push other people because I might alienate them or make them angry.		I can do my best and show others what can be done. I can be a positive catalyst for change.
I'm afraid my results will be wrong and this will show my incompetence.		If I don't try, I won't know what I can do.
I have trouble controlling my attention. I'm just too scattered to focus long enough to achieve results.		I can accomplish the task in small, manageable chunks.
If I'm swamped and overwhelmed, others are more likely to cut me a break. Because people see me as so busy, they do my work for me.		People don't like doing my work. They need me to carry my weight.
If I get results, I'll be finished. Then I'll just get more work to do.		I can move on to other things that interest or challenge me.

If you do think any of these statements, know that they are limiting beliefs; *all* they are is beliefs, not facts. Next to each one that you checked off, examine the alternative thoughts that would be healthier for you because they would unlock you and activate your energy toward results.

Now, when you hear yourself entertaining any of the thoughts on the left, think *Stop!* and consciously replace it with a thought from the right.

What if it isn't your thoughts that deter you, but rather the sheer difficulty of the work you need to accomplish? Try this next strategy.

Strategy Two: Prepare for Results

Projects and tasks feel the hardest at first blush. For most people, once you dedicate quality time to thinking about the project or task, you can envision what you're trying to achieve and how to achieve it in steps. Use the process found in the next tool to jump the hurdle of your resistance and fear of failure. Then, use Wendy's favorite tool, sticky-note planning (shown below), to organize the steps involved quickly and thoroughly.

✖ Tool: Up-Front Results Imaging

Purpose. This tool focuses you on the results you're aiming for—in rich detail, so you can create the prophecy you will then fulfill.

Method. Jot down the purpose you're trying to achieve by accomplishing the task or project. Jot down everything you already know about the desired results—the specifications that are obvious at this point.

- Read and reread what you wrote.
- Then shut your eyes, take a few deep breaths, and draw a picture in your mind's eye of the results you want, in rich detail. Really picture the finished product. Keep those eyes shut and push for the details. Flesh out your picture.
- Open your eyes, and jot down or somehow draw the imagery you drummed up around the results you want.
- Read and reread your imagery, and close your eyes one more time. This time, try to feel the feelings you'll have when you do achieve that result. Get into your success feelings, and think about the benefits of achieving these results.

Here's an example (Exhibit 6.2). Let's say you need to see to it that all of your employees attend a mandatory employee update. You receive the schedule of multiple sessions and get an instant headache at the thought of figuring out how to free up staff so they can attend. It's on your to-do list to figure out the schedule and make all the necessary arrangements. The mere thought of it feels overwhelming.

Exhibit 6.2. Example of Up-Front Results Imaging.

- *Jot down the purpose.* Make it possible for all of my staff to attend the employee update.

- *Take stock of what you already know.* The schedule of the updates and the schedule of my staff.

- *Picture the finished product.* The results you picture include staff members coming back from the update telling you they learned a lot and enjoyed the food.

- Picture components of the process of achieving these results:

  - A schedule in which you spread your staff across many sessions, so that you don't have to free too many people up at any one time

  - The names of the people who will attend each session

  - Decisions about which of those staff members require coverage and how you will provide it

  - A clear plan that shows who will order the replacement staff and when

  - The communication device you'll use to tell each staff member which update they need to attend

  - The feelings you'll have when you achieve the result. Pride, closure, a sense that you did the responsible thing (of getting your whole staff updated), and maybe a tad of relief that you avoided being on the list of "managers who didn't comply."

Try it yourself on a big project staring you down at this moment. Stare it down in your mind's eye and see if you can loosen up and get going on it.

Assuming you have the results in mind, the next step that catapults you forward is a plan, specifically one with subtasks, each of which is approachable and not overwhelming. Try this next tool to create project plans quickly, so you can move rapidly on them.

⚙ Tool: Sticky-Note Planning

Purpose. This tool organizes a complex project into subparts that make it easy for you to progress even if you only have a short bit of time.

Method. Get a 3" x 5" pad of sticky notes (Post-its). At the top of a blank wall, tape the results you want or need to achieve.

- Brainstorm all the subtasks or steps you'll need to perform to achieve these results. Don't write them down in a list. Instead, write down one step or subtask on each sticky note and spread them all out on a table.

- Look at the sticky notes and find the one you would need to do first, then second, then third. Move them to the wall to create a flowchart of the tasks to achieve the results you want. Since it's hard to get it right the first time, move the sticky notes around the wall until you get them in a sensible order.

- As you go along, you'll think of other subtasks. Write them on sticky notes too. Aim to fill the wall with your instructions for achieving the results.

- Decide which steps are milestones and mark them. Copy down what you've done on paper. Add responsibilities and timelines. Now you've got a plan, and you're hot to trot.

Even though having a clear conception of results and a plan for achieving them helps you overcome procrastination and gives you a jump-start, you're not home free yet. You must be able to control your *focus,* concentrating on each task without being distracted from it, or else it just stays on that to-do list endlessly. These days, focusing is no easy feat, because of the multiple demands on your attention.

Strategy Three: Focus, and Fend off Interruptions

Forget the clarity of the tasks, the obstacles, the barriers, the difficulty, and all the other factors. If you don't focus, you accomplish nothing or drag out the work over an intolerable period of time.

What stops people from focusing? Many things do, but we want to call your attention to one big force to reckon with: interruptions and how they seem to occur one after another, creating a chain of activities that absorb you but prevent you from making progress on what you intend to do. Here are some of the most notorious interruption situations, as well as an interruption control tool for each. Of course, it takes motivation on your part to use these devices, because you might allow interruption to avoid trying them out. But let's assume you really don't want to be consumed by interruption. Apply personal resolve and self-discipline and try some of the control tools suggested in Exhibit 6.3.

Exhibit 6.3. Interruption Control.

Situation	Interruption Control Tool
E-mail bleeps interrupt you and you're curious to see who's writing. You stop and read your e-mail very, very often.	Turn off the "notify" function. Pick a time of day when you will regularly read and respond . . . even twice a day is better than looking after every bleep.
You have no time for your own work, since you're so busy with meetings.	Create a committee of one. Call it something like the "Priorities Committee" and hold this time sacred for your priority work.
Your open-door policy causes people to pop in anytime, and you lose concentration.	Tell people that your closed door means "not now," and close it more often.
Others are not as busy as you, and they hang out in your office long past your tolerance point.	Go to their office for meetings. Then you can leave when you're finished.
You return calls when you know the person is unlikely to be in, because you're so busy.	This keeps the call on your to-do list and on someone else's. Pick a time when you're likely to reach the person; scheduling a time is even better. If you make it toward the end of the day, maybe they'll be eager to get home too.
Other?	

Share these ideas with your peers and make a pact to try to support each other and *not interrupt*. Respecting each other's time is a norm in a results-driven organization.

We've imagined the finish, we have some plans, and we're getting better at sticking to the tasks. But things still seem to take forever. What's the problem? Process, process, process. We two authors see well-intentioned managers trying desperately to get things done and feeling frustrated by endless processes. We are both committed to changing that with the folks we work with, and we believe there are solutions. The solutions entail embracing the importance of *speed*.

Strategy Four: Speed Up to Produce Results

Starting with the concept of small, frequent wins, Don Berwick, M.D., provides a terrific mental model for accomplishing improvements rapidly. He refers to this as "rapid cycle improvement" (Berwick, 1998).

You may already be steeped in some variation of the "plan-do-study-act" approach to continuous quality improvement. We found this model helpful for years, but we worried about its slowness. The fact is, quality improvement teams and many managers have spent gobs of time rigorously tackling a challenge large in scope, all with the intention to do a thorough, careful job of it. The rigor, the need to be both true to the data and scientific, caused many improvement teams to last months and months, sometimes years.

With rapid cycle improvement, you try things much sooner. You do a quick trial run and make course corrections, you try more things and make more course corrections, and on and on, rapid-fire. Exhibit 6.4 presents the basics of rapid cycle improvement as we see it.

Can you picture this working? Here's an example that might help. Wendy was working with an emergency department team to help them shorten the length of an ER visit. After learning about rapid cycle improvement, the team developed a series of short tests to try out. They asked, "What change can we complete by next Monday that will improve patient satisfaction with the length of an ER visit?" They focused on speedy trial ballooning of one idea after another.

Exhibit 6.4. Rapid Cycle Improvement.

- Set a goal.

- Figure out a simple, easy way to track progress on the goal. This method has to be one you can use daily.

- Figure out a series of tests or interventions that move you toward your goal. Keep them on a small scale, so you can try them quickly. Try it in one office, or with a group of volunteers, or in a simulation, or even with one customer. Any of these trials will cause you to learn about what happens and figure out "What next?" You may have to be creative to make a small test doable.

- Reduce the time frame for a single cycle from years, quarters, or months to days, hours, and minutes.

- Don't try to get everyone who is involved invested in the change or agreeing with it. Just try it.

- Gather useful data during each test.

- After it seems to work in one condition, try it over a growing range of conditions and people.

- Plan a few cycles at a time and then do one after the other.

To evaluate their trials, they instituted a two-question survey to monitor patient satisfaction:

1. How satisfied or dissatisfied were you with the time you spent receiving service in our ER?

2. On a four-point scale, how do you rate your satisfaction with your ER experience today?

They asked these questions of every patient or a family member; they kept running data they could eyeball every day. They posted a chart of results on the wall, so staff could see whether satisfaction with the length of visit was improving.

Here is a tool—a template—to help you work with your team using the rapid cycle improvement process (Exhibit 6.5).

Exhibit 6.5. Rapid Cycle Improvement: An Example.

Weekly Improvement Cycles to Increase ER Patient Satisfaction

Week 1　They attempted to alter patient and family expectations about the length of the visit. They tried out on five patients a new explanation, "Why Does It Take So Long?" They asked their two survey questions of these five patients to check results.

Week 2　They rearranged the schedules of two staff members, so that more people were available during peak times . . . to see if this staffing pattern reduced the time lag between procedures and tests for patients and reduced visit length.

Week 3　They rearranged certain equipment to make it easier for caregivers to access.

Week 4　They scripted a short explanation for the registrar to give to a patient and family during registration. It explained what would be done during the visit and how long it would take.

⚒ Tool: Rapid Cycle Improvement Planning

Purpose. This tool helps you create a plan for rapid cycle improvement related to an improvement goal.

Method. Pick an improvement goal that's important to your staff and customers. Form a small team of people with a stake in the improvement. Distribute the rapid cycle improvement plan below and fill it out.

- Brainstorm ways the group can get the first test up and running.

- Meet daily with the people doing the experiment to look at the data, talk about how it's going, and make *immediate* course corrections. Keep making the experiment more effective, modifying it every day as needed. Remind people that this isn't a scientific experiment. It's a rapid change process.

- Set weekly meeting times of your steering team to review the data, draw conclusions, and decide on the next test.

Rapid Cycle Improvement Plan

Our Goal Is:	What Is the Experiment?	Where and How Can We Try It?	In What Easy Way Can the Results Be Measured?	Who Will Make It Happen?	When Will It Start?
Test 1					
Test 2					
Test 3					
Test 4					
Test 5					

The next tool shows how simple the follow-up and follow-through process can be.

⚒ Tool: Daily Check-Ins

Purpose. This tool allows you to keep a close eye on each rapid cycle improvement test and decide daily how you're doing, as well as what to start doing, keep doing, or stop doing.

Method. Hold a daily huddle (ten minutes) with the stakeholders of the specific experiment in process. Two or three representatives are plenty.

Review the data for the previous day and the trend of all data collected so far. Ask, "What does this tell us?"

While focusing people on what to keep or change for the next day, ask:

- What's working? What should we keep doing, or do more of?
- What should we start doing? How should we adjust our approach?
- What should we stop doing?
- Get a clear fix on how to alter the experiment the next day.

Ta-daah! Say something that expresses both appreciation and excitement about continuing the experiment, for instance: "Hey, this is great. We're getting there! I'm excited about tomorrow, because I bet it's going to be a winner!"

Quick and dirty? Yes, that's the strength in this approach. You keep people in an action mode that produces rapid experiments, rapid results, and phenomenal learning along the way. You don't have to be a research scientist to make improvements. To get results, you need to try things, learn, try more things, and learn more. You *will* make improvements. Also, in the process you'll generate energy and excitement as people pull off improvements and make things better for patients.

Now, stretch your imagination a bit. Imagine what you could accomplish with that same ER team if they didn't have to do anything but work on solving the visit-length problem. Picture the improvements and results the group could make. If you are picturing it correctly, you have just conjured up a marathon meeting (see the next tool). Here, people work on one important issue at a time until they have solved it. They focus and they persist. They don't work on it in dribs and drabs, but in a scientific and focused way. This approach is great. Consider adopting it as you redesign work in your own areas.

Tool: Marathon Meeting

Purpose. This tool focuses attention on an important task so you can reach a solution quickly.

Method. Choose a process that *must* change, since keeping it as is is not a healthy option. Make sure you can get or have reliable data on your current process. Also make sure the people you assign to the project are invested in the outcome and want to find a better solution.

Here are the steps in the process:

1. *Define the scope.* Make sure everyone understands why the project is important and what the overall goals are in terms of outcome or result. Create a clear picture of the desired future state: "What do we want it to look like?"

2. *Define the current reality.* Observe and understand how things are now. Use data and observation to guide this education so that everyone understands what we are doing and why. You might shadow customers and staff, or use flowcharting and other data-collecting techniques. Pinpoint value-added and nonvalue-added steps in the process.

3. *Design the future state.* Create a map of the future. Use creative problem solving to help the group think out of the box. Focus on the ideas that help achieve your desired state. Design new work plans based on these ideas.

4. *Implement the desired state.* Begin implementing new plans and ideas. Use handholding and encourage people as needed.

5. *Monitor and learn.* Watch the process carefully. Correct your course as needed. Celebrate the learning, the effort expended, and the results.

What's the breakthrough here? This entire process may take three to five days, not weeks or months. Days! How? The people involved do nothing else. You heard it right. They only work on this project, and they work on it until they resolve it.

If you're rolling your eyes and saying, "How can I free people up for three days a week?" think again. Think about the time you and your peers spend in meeting after meeting going over the same issues, the same stories, achieving little. We know the marathon meeting may be a stretch, but we know too that it *saves* time in the long run.

To stay on this topic: a meeting can be a stopgap measure that paralyzes the result-getting process, or it can expedite results. Unfortunately, in most organizations meetings become the problem rather than the solution. Take heed and change this.

Strategy Five: Go After Results in Meetings

Let's say you're meeting with five colleagues about a project. Let's say that the average hourly rate of the group is $25. A two-hour meeting of the six of you costs your organization $25 per hour, times two hours, times six people, or $300, not counting the cost of opportunities or work each of you didn't pursue because you were at the meeting. The question is, Did the organization get $300 worth of value from the meeting?

The checklist in the next tool shows you the features of meetings that tend to be worth their weight in gold.

✖ Tool: Features of a Productive Meeting

Purpose. This tool helps you think through the components of a meeting that ensures results, so that you'll use your influence to bring these components into being.

Method. Take the checklist below to your next five meetings, and see how the group does on these features.

Productive Meeting Check

Feature	Appropriate Today?	Yes	No	Suggestions for Next Time
Person facilitating seemed prepared and focused.				
Meeting started on time, with little or no time spent schmoozing up front. Work began quickly.				
Early on, people shared completed tasks and results since last meeting; others gave them ta-daahs!				

Feature	Appropriate Today?	Yes	No	Suggestions for Next Time
By the end, nothing was fuzzy. The group nailed down agreements.				
Next steps, assignments, and time lines were clear.				
The group identified "invisible work" needed and parceled that out too.				
Someone took notes and agreed to distribute them within twenty-four hours.				

For a group with a pattern of producing few and far-between results, stick your neck out and show the members the tool, asking that people work together to make these meetings more productive by incorporating more of these features. Suggest further that someone serve as "navigator" at each meeting to ensure that the meeting *moves* and produces clear outcomes.

To push for results even more, here are two meeting variants that may help your group. They can give a whole team a push from passing time in meetings to making things happen:

- *The stand-up meeting.* This is a meeting in which people literally are not permitted to sit down. When you're standing, your energy is fully engaged. Also, the possibility that you will eventually get uncomfortable helps spur people to move quickly to make decisions, so you can all leave and sit down.
- *No meetings at all.* Then there's the "no meetings allowed" approach to meetings. Some organizations do not permit any morning meetings—no meetings before

2:00 P.M. This leaves time for working with staff and getting your other work done. If you can't be in meetings for all of those hours, you have time to do other important things. One organization we know allows no meetings at all. They emphasize taking personal responsibility for results and talking to the *individuals* associated with the work, not to groups in which too many people fade into the woodwork, bringing little to the party.

You're getting the picture, we suspect. Meetings devour time. Are they worth their weight in results? If not, get a grip on the meetings you hold and attend, and transform them into an opportunity for results. You will add to your value as a mover and shaker in your organization.

Strategy Six: Finish

Here you are, in an environment of multiple demands and diversions, with e-mail, snail mail, voice mail, staff members needing your attention, the phone, the fax machine, questions from your boss, questions from your customers, dozens of responsibilities, and many priorities. With so much on your plate, it is not easy to finish things and scratch them off your to-do list. You're waiting for information and answers. A canceled meeting slows you down. Circumstances change that throw a monkey wrench into your plans. Some projects and tasks take winding up and warming up, making you think the yield isn't worth the effort.

Results often fail to happen because the people working toward them stop short. Having done most of the work or prep, they just stop short. They fail to finish.

Our final advice to you in moving from busyness to a results-oriented mode is to get better at finishing (unless you're already good at it). By bringing things to closure, you feel accomplished and able to focus on other priorities without hearing the crackle of static from your overly cluttered mind and desk.

Consider this great way to finish those things left hanging and causing you and others to lose sleep—tasks that don't take long, but never seem to get done, such as cleaning a folder, filling the stapler, counting the inventory in the supply cabinet, taking down out-of-date items from the bulletin board, removing the waiting room magazines that are more than two years old, and the like.

⊗ Tool: The Finishing Frenzy

Purpose. This tool is useful for finishing a bunch of things, while letting you try out a technique you can use on occasion for this purpose.

Method. In a staff meeting, brainstorm tasks that are unfinished, tasks big and small. Write each task on a note card. Run through the cards. Getting group input, put on the card the time it's likely to take to finish that task.

- Select several tasks that will take only five minutes to do and that various people are capable of doing (as examples, returning a wheelchair to the ER, pulling outdated items off the bulletin board, cleaning up the dirty cups in the sink, making a sign showing people how to find the file room, and so on).

- Divvy up the five-minute tasks, asking each person to go do one in the next five minutes, reconvening afterward. When people reconvene, ask them to announce what they accomplished. Then ask how others react to this. They and you will probably be thrilled with the load of things accomplished.

- Take the rest of the cards and decide together where to put them so everyone with a few minutes can grab one and get something done. Perhaps create a "finishing board" or a "finishing box." Encourage people to help empty the board or the box by taking on tasks to get done.

- Now apply that same approach to your personal work. Make yourself a card for each of the many tasks you need or want to finish; include a time estimate. Grab one when you find yourself with a few minutes, thanks to an early lunch or a canceled meeting. Also consider scheduling "finishing school" as one of your regular meetings (with yourself) in which you take one of your finishing cards and do it.

- Next to your personal "to do" box, put another box called "did it!" As you complete a task, transfer the card to that box, and feel good as the cards pile up. You will see results galore.

Our Finish

To be a results-oriented manager, you have to think like one. When faced with the tough projects and challenges, you must prepare in ways that help you accomplish your work, that maintain your focus and control interruptions. You must respect the importance in this day and age of *speed* and move quickly, before needs and opportunities pass you by or problems overwhelm you and your staff and create additional problems for customers.

Do all you can to make meetings productive, not wasteful of people's precious time and energy. Be assertive, skillful, and persistent when you rely on someone's approval for something important you want to do. Make a habit of finishing things, so you can feel accomplished and move on.

But wait; there's one caveat. You can overdo your fervor for results and disrespect people in the process. We are not encouraging you to go after results *by any means necessary.* These days, because of the pressure many managers feel, they may place unreasonable demands on their colleagues and team. They push others beyond reasonable limits, with an eye to getting results. We are saying the ends are important, but we are not saying the ends justify the means. We encourage you to aim for results and engage in constructive strategies that help you achieve them, strategies that are in sync with your dearly held values.

Sometimes, people bypass discussion, consideration, or otherwise needed and reasonable processes because of their rush to finish or get results. When they do so, the ineffective process leaves wreckage along the way. If you are already a results-oriented manager and act that way, it might be more productive for you to consider how to strengthen your processes for getting results, so that everyone involved or affected feels good about the results, because they also feel good about the process.

Whether with staff, in meetings with colleagues, with your boss, or when you're trying to get things done with your door shut, determination, focus, planning, speed, self-discipline, leadership, and use of processes that value others are all required to behave as an effective results-oriented manager. The good news is that the dedicated effort this requires of you yields an enormous return on your investment.

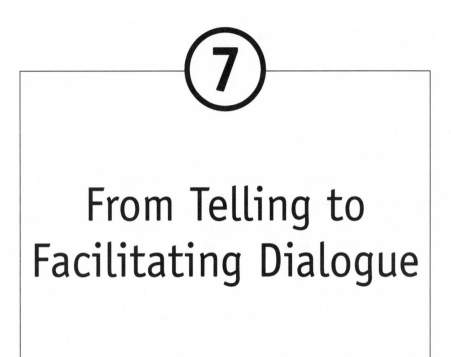

From Telling to Facilitating Dialogue

Are you familiar with the manager who does most of the talking, who tells people what they are supposed to do and what they need to know, communicating in a telling manner? These days, this one-way-only communication style stunts the group's energy, creativity, learning, and results. Instead, imagine a work culture where information, perceptions, feelings, and ideas flow freely; where people express themselves and respect each other's viewpoints; where all team members, colleagues, and customers speak up for the good of the team and the mission. This is a culture of engagement. It is a culture that mobilizes people. They have their say, and the group benefits from the many and varied perspectives and talents of each individual.

A Revealing Look in the Mirror

True or False?	True	False
1. I am uncomfortable with conflict and controversy in groups.	___	___
2. As far as communication goes, I believe that my main job is to give people information.	___	___
3. I try to encourage dialogue in our meetings, but the angry or resistant types tend to take over.	___	___
4. I don't ask my staff or colleagues what they think when the outcomes and decisions are out of their control.	___	___
5. I don't urge people to speak up if I think it will make them uneasy or uncomfortable.	___	___
6. I work hard to create an atmosphere of openness and trust in all of my relationships.	___	___
7. I actively try to manage rumors and misinformation within my team.	___	___
8. I understand that when I open the group up to real dialogue, I may hear things that make me uncomfortable.	___	___
9. I deliberately use a variety of communication methods, because there are a variety of learners with different needs.	___	___
10. I make sure everyone in my group shares responsibility for giving and getting information.	___	___

If you answered false to the first five questions and true to the remaining five, you know the importance of open, honest dialogue with the various stakeholders within your team, throughout your organization, among your customers, and in your community. Also, you see yourself as responsible for facilitating this dialogue. You recognize your critical role in creating an environment that encourages openness and trust, since you want your team and your organization to benefit from the ideas, engagement, and support of your customers, colleagues, and staff. You don't see yourself as the sole source of important information but instead expect everyone on your team to share responsibility for gathering and sharing information.

It's a New Day

These days, every manager needs to dedicate energy and time to building a work culture where information flows freely, where people express and respect each other's opinions. We also want everyone on the team to share responsibility for not only maintaining great communication but also tapping the entire team's thinking to produce optimal results. But it is not easy to move from a telling style to one of active engagement and dialogue.

Those of us groomed in a hierarchical organization typically have experience with the manager who relies heavily on telling as the predominant communication style. We daresay this continues to be the prevailing style in many health care organizations. This manager feels committed to communicating, but the communication stops at conveying information. The manager says, "Here are our goals. Here are our plans. Here's what our methods will be." The boss tells employees what they need to know; the manager tells employees to tell customers what the rules are and what they can expect. Managers expect to be told by their higher-ups what they're supposed to do. Telling, telling, telling.

Back when health care and our world were simpler, when people accepted authority without question, telling as a communication style appeared to work fine. One-way communication was a norm that fit the culture. Although opportunities for dialogue and discourse may have been few and far between, people didn't expect them either. Managers did not ask people to share their opinions, react, or respond. Managers expected them to listen, digest, and accept the information at hand.

Many people (especially parents) yearn for the good old days when people seemed to respect authority and accept being told how things would be. No more. It is much more the norm today that employees want their voices to be heard and their views and ideas respected. Many want to participate actively in designing services; identifying and solving problems; setting goals; and influencing, if not making, decisions. Those who do not are a concern to us. Perhaps their silence reflects a feeling of being disaffected, passive, or detached from our team and the buzz of organizational life. In any case, we miss out on their thinking.

We say, engage people when you're with them. Draw them in; hear them out. Make it easy for them to express themselves and react to what others are saying. It is vital today for people to understand that great communication is critical to a healthy system, and making that happen is everyone's responsibility. This is a shift, and we managers need to lead the charge.

Take a Look

Managers who tell handle everyday situations differently than do managers who facilitate dialogue. Their results tell the tale.

Rodney

Rodney has inherited employees who actively resist getting involved. They often don't show up for meetings, claiming, "Why bother? No one cares what we think." When they do attend, they don't say what they're thinking. His employees are a bit more open when Rodney talks with them individually, but he still has a hard time getting them to open up, ask questions, or share their ideas. He's at a loss about what to do.

Operating with a telling style, Rodney does nothing to change the dynamic in his group and continues one-way communication, to no avail. He rationalizes, "That's the way these people are, and there's little I can do to change it." Secretly, he is most comfortable with one-way communication and feels anxiety at the thought of dialogue and controversy. With dialogue, he knows he can't control what people say, and he's not confident he can handle whatever might come up. Rodney has a long history of discomfort with controversy; faced with it, he jumps in quickly with a resolution.

If Rodney were to abandon his practice of telling and embrace the role of facilitator of dialogue, he would handle this situation with his team differently. Understanding that dialogue is important and facilitation of dialogue involves skills, he can ask a colleague to coach him to become a more effective facilitator with his team. Also, he talks with folks in his organization's training department to see whether opportunities are available to help him enhance his communication and facilitation skills. Most important, he tells his staff that he wants them to participate more and that he plans to work on his skills, so he can make it easier for them.

Susan

Susan manages a large group with people working on all three shifts. She is finding it difficult to keep everyone involved and informed; she feels that, no matter what she does, people always say, "No one told us that" or "Who made *that* decision?" Susan finds herself spending a lot of her precious time clearing up rumor and misunderstanding.

Steeped in a telling style of communication, Susan feels that rumor and misunderstanding are inevitable in organizational life, and that she just needs to learn to live with them. She also believes that staff use "No one told me this" as an excuse to disengage, and that no matter what she does these people will hear what they choose to hear. She keeps communicating the way she always has.

If Susan were to switch to a style of facilitating dialogue, she would think and act differently. As a dialogue facilitator, she takes pains to find ways to communicate with the evening, night, and weekend staff. She makes sure to communicate with people face-to-face, not just in writing. She thinks through what she wants to discuss and plans a variety of ways to expedite dialogue. She knows she needs to share important information repeatedly, thus creating more than one opportunity for her team to discuss and react. She also communicates to her team that they are to stay informed as a job expectation. She talks with people about the consequences for the group when people don't take advantage of opportunities to stay up to date.

Daniela

Daniela has a couple of naysayers on her team. They frequently complain, turn meetings into a gripe session, and have the effect of stirring up their coworkers. Their coworkers tire of it, but they don't feel comfortable challenging this outspoken subgroup. To make matters worse, the naysayers usually buzz in the parking lot, where they twist whatever people have said during a meeting. Daniela believes that this group is fueling negative feelings and a morale problem throughout the team.

Managing naysayers is never easy, but it's even harder for managers with a telling style. As a telling manager, Daniela feels powerless to control the negativity in the group and backs off entirely. She avoids holding regular meetings and, on the rare occasions when she convenes the group, does all the talking, hoping to crowd out the naysayers' naysaying. She doesn't address their behavior or its effect on the group. Needless to say, morale does not improve.

As a manager who facilitates dialogue, Daniela thinks and behaves differently. First of all, she realizes that the negative energy in the group won't go away without some intervention on her part. She realizes that, no matter how uncomfortable it may be, she must address it. She decides to raise her concerns frontally in the group and plans how to do so constructively, avoiding blame that creates even more divisiveness. Her main message: "I'm asking your help in building a climate where we make room for everyone's thoughts and ideas. I'm concerned that we're losing out on what some people think by allowing a few individuals to do the lion's share of the talking. I want everyone to have room to participate." Daniela invites the group to identify ground rules for group discussion, rules that afford space and support for everyone's contributions.

Bill

Bill's board and executive team have just completed a strategic planning process in which they did not solicit employee input. Now, employees are being invited to attend a presentation where they will hear the results. Along with other managers, Bill is disappointed that the planning process made no room for their perspectives or suggestions. His employees are going to the presentation to hear the plan as a fait accompli.

As a telling manager, he schedules his employees to attend, telling them beforehand, "I want you to go, because this new plan is important for you to know."

As a manager committed to dialogue and himself disappointed that he had no input into the planning process, Bill prepares his people differently. He says, "I'm really looking forward to all of us knowing the strategic direction and main initiatives our board and executive team believe are the key to our future. Please attend with an ear to where our organization is heading, and then let's get together to share our reactions and talk about how we can contribute. We have a great opportunity to develop our plans so that they help us move in the desired direction."

In advance, Bill's people know they have a chance for dialogue about the implications of the plan. Bill engages his team in dialogue even though higher-ups in his organization did not engage or involve him and his fellow directors.

What Worries You?

Becoming a dialogue facilitator is not easy if you have a history of both being told by your boss and telling your team. Which of these concerns or feelings strike a chord with you?

Do you feel unsettled or anxious when you don't know where a conversation or dialogue is going? Managers tell us that their greatest fear about facilitating dialogue is that it will get out of control. It feels risky to encourage it, because people might say or do things that the manager does not know how to handle. It seems easier and safer to keep a lid on things and just tell folks what to do and how things will be.

Do you worry that, by inviting dialogue, you are leading people on? Certainly, there are times when a decision has been made and is not negotiable, when people have to be told what to do. Some managers want to curb dialogue in such a situation. They fear that people will think the decision reversible. They also worry about challenges to their authority in ways they don't know how to handle.

Do you feel anxious that people who want to have their own way will bog down the discussion and create an impasse? True, some people are not satisfied unless they have it their way. They hear what they want to hear, ignoring whatever does not fit their version of the truth. If you give them an inch, they'll take a mile. Better not to give them even an inch.

Do you think dialogue takes more time and patience than you and your team have to spare? Some managers hesitate to engage people in discussion because they perceive it as endless and pointless unless it results in a clear plan and decision. They don't value process. In their eagerness or even impatience to get things done, they think neither they nor their team members should be wasting time sharing thoughts and feelings.

Do you feel like a failure when you invite dialogue and people do not respond? Some managers feel ineffective when they ask a question and no one says a word. Because this makes them so uncomfortable, they stop asking questions and instead resort to telling. The fact is, since most of our organizations are hierarchical, many employees are afraid to speak or challenge authority and the status quo unless it is clear that this is a safe thing to do.

Do you prefer to avoid challenge, controversy, and confrontation? Many managers and nonmanagers find conflict unsettling and something to avoid at all cost, in and beyond the realm of their work. When facilitating dialogue, it is possible for conflict to result. This makes some people avoid it altogether so as not to take the risk.

Encouraging openness, direct communication, and discussion is challenging at best. Yet the price we pay by avoiding it is high. People are disengaged, resistant, or resentful if they have not had a voice or a chance to influence what is happening around them. This disengagement, resistance, and resentment inhibits the process of change, generating negative vibes with customers and hurting the team's productivity and spirit.

What Do You Stand to Gain?

Your customers, employees, organization, and you yourself benefit when employees are actively engaged in sharing their ideas, participating in decisions, reacting to information and options, and questioning.

- If you don't permit employees and colleagues to express themselves, if you don't invite them into the process by sparking dialogue, *you pay the price.* As we move further away from the age when authority reigned, people want and expect to participate. If they don't have that chance, many become disheartened, perhaps reacting by becoming passive, apathetic, resistant, or resentful in your presence. They unplug, and you lose their energy and commitment. What happens outside of your presence? They save their dialogue for the meeting-after-the-meeting. They have their say in an informal, vociferous hallway or lunchroom conversation in which the staff members who sat quietly in your meeting not only find their voices but also find people who listen. For better or for worse, people then share with each other what they heard and how they feel about it and about you, and you have no chance to respond, benefit, or know what they're thinking. Dialogue, in contrast to one-way communication, draws people in as stakeholders in your decisions and plans.

- *When people engage in dialogue, they hear and retain more information.* Unlike one-way communication, dialogue pushes people into an active mode. If you communicate a pile of important information without getting feedback about what people have heard, understood, and thought, they are likely to have the information that you think is so important go in one ear and out the other.

- *In dialogue, the group comes to share responsibility for communication.* The weight does not rest entirely on you. This is a relief, just as it becomes a learning opportunity for your team.

- *Negativity in groups takes its toll on staff morale and spirit.* You can influence this through dialogue. When you generate dialogue, you give people airtime and an arena for expressing their concerns openly. This gives you and other group members the chance to transform what would otherwise be persistent negativity into constructive communication.

- *Skilled in dialogue, you become a valuable member of the leadership team.* You also, by the way, become more marketable. You can help promote dialogue with customers and colleagues in other departments and teams.

- *You capitalize on everyone's thinking.* There is simply too much to do, and there are too many problems to solve to generate all of the know-how and ideas yourself. Through dialogue, you unleash the thinking and diverse perspectives of your whole team. When you admit that you don't have all the answers, team members help. Given room to contribute, they do. The more diverse your team is, the more the group and the organization benefit from multiple perspectives. As you involve others in the process, you yield better answers and better results.

• *Open, honest communication builds trust in you; you gain credibility.* Many employees are suspicious of leaders, not convinced that the leaders have their interests at heart. By facilitating dialogue with your folks, you replace *we-they* with *we.*

What Can You Do? How Can You Do It?

If you've grown up in an atmosphere of being told, you may find it hard to become a facilitator of dialogue, unless you've had the opportunity to develop this strength through reading, mentoring, team participation, or educational programs. If you see the benefits of facilitating dialogue and want to build your skill repertoire, you can proceed by pursuing four strategies (Exhibit 7.1) and trying out the tools we relate to each one.

Exhibit 7.1. Strategies to Move from "Telling" to Facilitating Dialogue.

Strategy one: Think like a facilitator of dialogue.

Strategy two: Create a safe container.

Strategy three: Build important dialogues into everyday life.

Strategy four: Become a skillful catalyst of dialogue.

The first strategy helps you adopt beliefs that prompt you to facilitate dialogue. This entails addressing the fears and concerns triggered by considering this shift. It also prompts you to consider your commitment to becoming a manager who invites and welcomes dialogue.

The second strategy involves creating an atmosphere, or safe container, that promotes open discussion among individuals and groups. This involves using techniques to ensure widespread participation, developing ground rules for communication, and enforcing these ground rules.

The third strategy identifies the content and key messages of dialogues we think are critical in today's environment, in the hope that you plan for these dialogues and build them into your routines. It goes further by helping you trigger a real exchange of views in the kind of top-down communication that in most organizations tends to be an I-speak-you-listen experience.

The final strategy helps you become a skilled catalyst, helping people talk with each other respectfully and productively. It also helps you prepare to handle sticky situations when you feel a discussion is veering off course, and you know you need to intervene to return it to a productive direction.

Strategy One: Think Like a Facilitator of Dialogue

Do your thoughts make it hard for you to depart from a style of telling? Consider these concerns, typical of managers accustomed to a telling approach to communication.

- *"Dialogue takes time."* Up front, it takes more time than telling. Down the pike, it takes less time. It does take time to encourage response and discussion. But think about what you hope to achieve every time you do share information. Is the point to impart information, or to make sure that people digest and embrace it? When you engage people in dialogue, you spend more time up front and less time later, because people are on the same page and working with you, not against you. What really consumes time are the consequences of misunderstanding and resistance. Whether with your team or colleagues from other departments, you have to handle this endlessly if people have not felt respected by your involving them.
- *"I need to be in control."* Many leaders fear losing control if they encourage conversation and people react unpredictably or disturbingly. Even highly skilled facilitators share this fear. They learn, however, that most of us operate under an *illusion* of control. We can control the moment, but we can't control other people's thoughts and responses after the moment has passed. People will talk, they will share their concerns or ideas in some way to someone, whether this happens in our presence or not. Can you see how much better it is for you and your partners if people share their thoughts and feelings directly? The good news is that the more you learn about ways to facilitate and encourage dialogue, the more in control you feel. An alternative understanding might be "I can't always be in control, and that's OK," or "I can learn ways to effectively guide dialogue. I can learn how to intervene when it is becoming unproductive without shutting people down."

Leaders who encourage dialogue believe that they are doing so because dialogue is healthy and important. They realize that they may have to learn new skills, but they know that with time and practice they can do so. And they want to.

To become more of a dialogue facilitator, consider the thoughts you have that help and hinder you from achieving this. This first tool helps you identify arguments you can use on yourself to push you in the direction of dialogue.

Tool: How Do I Benefit?

Purpose. This tool helps you identify the benefits of fostering open, honest dialogue within your team.

Method. Go to a quiet place where you will not be disturbed. Put work aside and make sure that you can have a few moments for reflection.

- Close your eyes and imagine that you are in one of your staff meetings, but this meeting is the way you have always hoped your meetings would be. People are talking and sharing ideas. Questions are being asked, and the group is responding. Continue thinking about the interaction and dialogues that are taking place in your ideal meeting.
- Open your eyes, and take a few moments to reflect on this experience. Jot down some of the things that you thought about in this ideal fantasy, things that you would love to see happen in your own meetings.
- Now think about how you felt during this experience, and think about how staff seemed to feel and respond in your ideal. Think about the benefits if this type of meeting were not a fantasy, but a reality in your group. What would be the benefits for you, your staff, your customers, and your organization?

Becoming a skilled facilitator is a lifelong journey. We both have devoted years to learning more and better ways to enhance our own skills, and neither of us will ever feel finished. We are all a work in progress. Both of us are fortunate because we have had wonderful mentors and role models who enabled us to observe great facilitation skills in action and develop our own skills with feedback and coaching.

Sounds simple, but when it happens—when someone facilitates conversation, bringing people together to share their ideas nonthreateningly—it only looks easy. You and I know it isn't true. Use this next tool to visualize the difference between someone you know who facilitates dialogue well and someone else who has the opposite effect of shutting people down.

✖ Tool: I Know It When I See It

Purpose. This tool helps you see the difference in behavior and impact of a manager who you know facilitates dialogue well, compared to another manager who gets in the way of constructive interchange.

Method. Choose two individuals. The first should be someone you find easy to talk to. We'll call this person the "opener." Conversation flows easily, and you feel free to share your thoughts and ideas. You are comfortable with the person and the relationship.

- The second person, "the closer," should be someone with whom you have a troubled relationship. You feel uncomfortable sharing your views, and you hesitate to be honest and open with this person.

- Think about a conversation you had with each person. Jot down your memories of both conversations, including the things you and the other person did or said. Look over your notes and think about the difference between the two exchanges. What does the opener do that makes you feel comfortable and encourages you to open up? Conversely, what does the closer do to discourage openness on your part and cause you to shut down?

- Consider committing yourself to becoming a skilled facilitator. Articulate in your own mind the impact you want to have on people.

Use the information you got from the previous exercise to help you become more aware of what you do and say in conversation with other people. You will discover that unlike the telling manager, the facilitative manager does many things to open up dialogue, starting with creating conditions that encourage open exchange.

Strategy Two: Create a Safe Container

The dictionary describes a facilitator as one who makes things easier. For our discussion, a facilitator is one who creates an environment—a safe container—that encourages people to open up and share their views and concerns. Many people are hesitant to talk in groups. Some fear that others will judge them. Some worry about saying something others will see as dumb. Still others are shy and clam up. Most people are likely to talk if you do something to ease their way into the discussion.

Successful facilitators understand how to engage the group initially, getting everyone to talk in an atmosphere of support. They also work with their team to establish ground rules for constructive team meetings and share responsibility for enforcing the rules. Also, they consciously develop and demonstrate behavior that aids dialogue and avoid behavior that inhibits it. Let's look at how you can help to create a safe container for dialogue.

To begin, here are a few tried-and-true approaches dialogue facilitators use to draw everyone into discussion initially:

- Pose the discussion question to the group, but ask them to discuss it with one other person first before talking in the whole group.

- Ask people to talk in a small, safe-feeling group, brainstorming or figuring out a point the small group wants to pose to the whole group. This allows safety in numbers for the individual reticent about speaking up in the bigger group.

- Ask participants to jot down a few notes or fill out a short set of questions before you attempt to trigger discussion in the larger group.

- Place specific topics or feelings to be discussed around the room, and let people gather around the one that attracts them. Ask the "we like . . ." groups to chat before inviting dialogue in the whole group.

- Ask small groups to plan and lead a topic for group discussion.

Sometimes dialogue happens without anyone doing anything to trigger it. More often than not, it is made to happen by design. The tools presented here are great dialogue triggers. The first two help you set the stage for interaction in your team meetings. Both are quick and easy to do, and they show that you value what people are thinking and feeling.

✖ Tool: How Are You Feeling?

Purpose. This tool helps people see where others are coming from.

Method. Put these words on a sheet of paper, and ask people to circle the words that best describe their feelings about a particular issue or event:

Motivated

Interested

Hopeful

Skeptical

Worried

Confused

Excited

Enthusiastic

Stressed

Tired

Then ask each person to talk to a partner about word choice.

Let partners discuss how they would like to feel and what that would take—from them, from the group, and from the leader. Invite reports to the whole group.

Here's another dialogue starter, "What's on Top?" that helps people spill whatever is on their minds. Without asking for these thoughts and feelings, people keep them under wraps or hold back. When people are hiding their feelings rather than expressing them, this affects their behavior and the discussion, usually negatively.

Tool: What's on Top? (Scott, 1996a)

Purpose. This tool eases people into group dialogue.

Method. Ask folks to think about something that is on their mind at the moment. It does not need to be work-related, although it could be. It should be whatever is going on at the moment.

Begin with one person sharing what's on top of his or her mind. Go around the room or table until everyone has had a turn who wants one, but allow people the option of passing and jumping in later. Whip around, giving everyone a turn. Ask people to avoid questions or comments about what someone else said until the very end.

A manager we know asked his group, "What's on top?" and a member of the group shared that her husband had just been diagnosed with cancer. This gave the team an opportunity to offer understanding and support. It also gave this woman the chance to explain her withdrawn behavior. You know that people bring more than their bodies to a meeting. When you give people an opportunity to connect and facilitate emotions, they will open up. If you want your team members to share what is on their mind, actively encourage them to do so.

Once you have encouraged people in discussion using tools like these, you and the group should continue to encourage openness and participation and actively avoid discouraging it. How? By creating a common vision and clear ground rules for team interaction. Group members can then refer to the rules if behavior gets out of hand, saying, "Wait! Remember our agreement!" It is a concrete way to monitor group interaction that goes a long way toward creating a safe environment for dialogue. Here's a simple process.

⚒ Tool: Setting Ground Rules

Purpose. This tool helps your team establish ground rules that support communication, not discourage it.

Method. Ask your group to think about behavior on the part of others that helps or hinders trust, participation, and open discussion.

Capture these thoughts on a flip chart or wallboard. Ask the group to cluster the comments into a few categories. For instance, ground rules might include:

- Listen to what others are saying.

- Check out what people mean; don't make assumptions.

- Respect others by coming on time, prepared to work.

- Support others' ideas and suggestions. State what you agree with before you offer alternatives.

Help the group build on these ideas by talking about occasions on which they see people demonstrating the behavior and the impact it has on the group. End the discussion by identifying together one or two behaviors that people realize they must adopt for the sake of rich and uninhibited dialogue.

By asking your team to become aware of behavior and commit to demonstrating the helpful and abandoning the negative, you engage the group in creating the conditions for constructive dialogue. But it doesn't end here. Team members have to hold themselves and others accountable to these agreements. This won't be easy, and we think the first step is yours. Set the stage by anticipating and preventing group problems whenever possible. But if you haven't managed to prevent destructive behavior from occurring, you must then intervene to keep the discussion constructive. Individual problems left unchecked turn into group problems.

Here's a simple case. What if you have naysayers on your team who tend to cut people off and jump on other people's ideas? You should intervene, dealing with it directly for the sake of preserving the safe container for dialogue. In Exhibit 7.2, we present some intervention options to consider when dialogue becomes destructive.

Exhibit 7.2. Intervention Options When Dialogue Becomes Destructive.

- *Discuss the rules in the group.* Remind the whole group of their own ground rules. Ask them to think about when and how people are demonstrating this behavior. This is helpful when many individuals need to look at their behavior, but it is less helpful when one or two individuals are violating the group norms. In our case study, discussion of the ground rules allows people to talk about their feelings when other people cut them off.

- *Discuss the rules and the behavior outside of the group.* After the meeting, take aside the individuals who are disrupting the dialogue and remind them gently about the group norms. Note what you observed and ask them to catch themselves in future discussion. This direct approach gives you a chance to find out more about what might be going on for these people. Are they unplugged, annoyed, or what? Or do they unintentionally interfere with group discussion? Sometimes people are blind to their own behavior and don't see their impact unless confronted directly.

- *Discuss the behavior in the group.* Bring up issues about individual behavior in the group. Since this can be threatening, we suggest doing so only after you've tried the first two options. It's the most direct, but the riskiest, approach. It works best once your group becomes accustomed to giving each other feedback and examining their behavior.

Strategy Three: Build Important Dialogues into Everyday Life

This third strategy helps you create dialogue around recurrent topics important to your group's life. No doubt, in your role, you are expected to communicate piles of information to your staff. There are indeed some important topics that staff deserve to know about so they can invest in the organization's goals and be attentive to rules, news, plans, and progress. Also, they deserve to be told this information by you, since as manager you are their lifeline to the sources of this information.

Exhibit 7.3 suggests what information is important to share periodically.

Exhibit 7.3. Important Topics for Regular Communication.

Information about the big picture (mission, vision, values, and plans of the organization)

Challenges facing the organization

Information about customer satisfaction, compliments, and complaints

Service stories and recognition

Changes in the department and organization

Departmental plans

Updates about staffing and other resources

Policy updates

Budget issues

New technology and tools available

Problems and sticky situations needing solutions

Managers who are effective communicators use a variety of methods to communicate, including face-to-face meetings with individuals or groups, phone calls, broadcast voice mail, e-mail, posted memos, newsletters, letters, weekly updates, bulletin boards, and the like. The challenge is, no matter which method you use, to somehow trigger dialogue instead of keeping the communication one-way.

How do you make dialogue happen around the important topics that we're used to communicating in a one-way, I-tell-you-listen form? Complicating matters even further, how do you do this when you have employees working on different shifts or at several locations?

E-mail, Internet chat rooms, and intranets have created great tools for interaction in writing. If you and your staff have access to them, learn how to enter questions into these media and how to solicit answers from your staff. Better yet, learn how to enable a multiparty conversation by way of a chat room, if your organization has a Website or intranet.

Ask a few members of your team to interview others in the group on a hot topic. Post the responses on the bulletin board.

Hold a five-minute sound-off meeting on a sticky issue. Hold this short gathering several times during the day (and night) so many people can attend. Again, post the results and comments.

Also, if you have staff working day and night seven days a week, you can facilitate dialogue without even holding meetings by using the next tool.

✖ Tool: Mural Dialogue

Purpose. This tool engages staff in dialogue when they can't talk to each other face to face.

Method. Hang a huge strip of shelf paper on a wall. Post information you want to communicate and a question related to that information. For instance, if you have information about a new policy, let's say on patient confidentiality, post the policy on one end of the mural and ask, "Where and how do we have problems with patient confidentiality? What can we do about them?"

Hang pens and markers from the mural and invite people to enter comments, questions, pictures, or whatever addresses the question at hand. Encourage people to sign their entries so others know who they are listening to.

Meet with staff on all three shifts and explain the mural dialogue approach to them, framing the first question and asking them to talk to their colleagues from other shifts by entering comments on the mural. Change the paper every so often.

Hopefully, these tools and tips expand your repertoire as communicator and facilitator of dialogue. But remember, you don't have to be the only one to share information. Giving and receiving information is everyone's responsibility. Unless you can help your folks share responsibility for communication, they will continue to say, "Nobody ever tells me anything!"

Our final tool in this section is a way to guide your group in taking responsibility for sharing information and talking about it in meetings, without your having to be the sole facilitator.

⚒ Tool: Monthly "Bits" (Scott, 1996c)

Purposes. This tool affords consistency and continuity in your regular meetings, covers a range of topics in a relatively short period of time, and helps staff take responsibility for portions of the meeting.

Method. Divide your monthly staff meeting into discrete sections or "bits." These can be:

- People: things that individual team members have accomplished this month

- Plans: upcoming plans or improvements

- Problems: those needing to be discussed from a customer or staff perspective

- Personal sharing: learning or insights people have had during the month

- Progress: the status of any projects or teams

- Projects: those needing to be initiated or reviewed

After each meeting, post the notes from each section so that people who weren't there get the bits. Post a fresh "bit board," and let people sign up during the month for the bits that they want to discuss.

Assign a bit to an individual or team. These people collect from you and others the hot topics to be discussed under their bit and facilitate the dialogue at the next meeting.

Strategy Four: Become a Skillful Catalyst of Dialogue

We have saved the best for last. Back at the beginning of this chapter, we asked you to think of two individuals who encouraged or discouraged dialogue. You were asked to consider the specific things these people did to set the stage, to open people up. This was not an easy exercise, as sometimes it may be difficult to pinpoint behavior. Sometimes it's just a feeling you get from a person that makes you think, *This person cares about what I have to say.* Nonetheless, there are behaviors that do make a difference.

Here are some of our favorite promoters and killers of dialogue, knowledge of which can help you facilitate effective communication (Exhibit 7.4). Take these tips with you to your next several meetings. Consciously follow these suggestions, notice the effects, and we're sure you'll be encouraged.

We hope that, by considering and trying out these tips, you'll become more conscious of your behavior and its effects. Further these insights by inviting a colleague to observe you and give you feedback in one of your staff meetings. Give them these tips ahead of time, so they will watch the relevant behaviors on your part.

The suggestions might seem awkward at first, but with practice you become more aware of what you do and don't do—and skilled at getting people talking.

Exhibit 7.4. Dialogue Promoters and Killers.

1. *Ask open-ended questions, particularly those starting with "what."* Pose questions that require thinking and more than a yes or no answer. Questions that begin with "what" are particularly useful in promoting dialogue. For instance:

   What concerns do you have?

   What patterns do you see in these complaints?

   What is your reaction to these changes?

2. *Respond in ways that keep the conversation going and flowing.* Respond positively to all contributions, without necessarily agreeing or disagreeing. Show appreciation for people who participate; this will encourage others to join in. Nod your head as you listen. Say "uh huh." Maintain eye contact. Appear reflective. Appreciate what people are saying with "thanks," "yes," "great," "right on," and other reactions that encourage their participation, without necessarily agreeing or disagreeing with what they're saying.

   Probe. Ask for more. For example, "Tell me more about that." Or "What's an example of that, so we'll get a better idea of what you're thinking?"

3. *Make connections to create a flow of ideas and encourage people to build on and relate to what others have said.* Connect the different points people make: "Again," "As Jim has been saying in another way," and so on.

Exhibit 7.4. (continued)

Refer to what people have said previously. For instance, "Joe mentioned it before," "Just as Mary said yesterday," "Susan, you helped us see this today." This again is a form of positive reinforcement.

4. *Avoid dialogue-killers.* Don't judge or evaluate every response. If you say "right" or "good" after some people's responses, those who don't receive that response from you feel as if their contributions are being negatively received. This shuts people down.

   Don't repeat, comment, or build on every person's remarks. Avoid a pattern of dialogue in which a person says something, then you respond, another person says something, and you respond. If you keep drawing attention back to yourself after every comment by another person, folks stop addressing each other and focus their comments on you— that is, if they continue making comments at all.

   Don't disagree outright. If you're the boss, you have disproportionate power in the group. In that case, instead of disagreeing ask, "What do others think about this?" Or "Do others see this the same way?" This invites others into the conversation.

   Don't ignore responses. Acknowledge responses, even if they don't add a great deal to the conversation.

   Don't let people go on and on. Some participants will talk endlessly. If you don't intervene, the rest of the group will disengage. Help the talker come to the point. For instance, "You're saying several things. Help us see your main point." Or "Thanks. Now I'm curious to hear what other people think."

5. *When dialogue is dwindling or you need to draw it to a close, summarize and identify next steps.* For instance: "We'll talk more about this on Tuesday, starting, I suggest, with this question. . . . Please think about that and we can discuss it further then." Or "So, we've agreed to . . . Now we can. . . . "

A Diatribe About Dialogue

Gone are the days when employees sit still and smile in the face of one-way communication or telling. They want to be involved, not put to sleep by being talked at incessantly. You have an opportunity to shine as a manager by learning how to ask open-ended questions and encouraging, not hampering, dialogue.

It would be ironic to end this chapter on facilitating dialogue by telling you even more. So, instead we'll close with three questions that we hope spur your thinking and dialogue with your colleagues.

First, to what extent do you get dialogue to happen among your team? Why so much, or why not?

Second, in what situations would you like to foster dialogue at work?

Third, what ideas are you thinking of applying to make these dialogues happen?

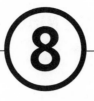

From Protecting Turf to Building Relationships

Although managers may not consciously choose to protect their turf above all, many hang on to this pattern tenaciously, as a survival strategy. In today's environment, the successful leader realizes the importance of moving from mastery within the span of direct influence to stepping out of the comfort zone to build collaborative relationships. Because of the complexity and interdependency of functions and services, there are simply too many challenges and opportunities that demand partnering among stakeholders and open dialogue about how best to pursue shared goals.

A Revealing Look in the Mirror

True or False?	True	False
1. I try to stay focused on my work and not get involved in personal issues.	____	____
2. I do whatever it takes to make sure my team gets the resources they want.	____	____
3. I focus on my own areas and try not to be concerned with what is going on in other departments.	____	____
4. I avoid putting myself in situations where conflict might occur.	____	____
5. Some people are just difficult to work with, and it isn't worth it to me to get involved.	____	____
6. I know that my success depends on the cooperation and support of other people and groups.	____	____
7. I avoid blaming and finger-pointing when things go wrong.	____	____
8. I try to work well with colleagues for the good of our customers.	____	____
9. Being a great team player means putting myself in other people's shoes.	____	____
10. I dedicate time to building teamwork and harmonious relationships among my staff.	____	____

If you responded false to the first five statements and true to the last five, you understand the importance of working collaboratively with others, for the sake of your customers, your staff, and your own effectiveness. Relationship-oriented managers address personal issues whenever these issues affect the quality and approach to work. They respect people's feelings and needs, without dismissing them as irrelevant or inappropriate. They engage in direct communication and confrontation when required to ease strain in a relationship. They recognize that success rests on cooperation and teamwork, and that it is their responsibility to *earn* them.

Perhaps you are lucky enough to work in an environment that actively supports strong relationships with colleagues and people outside of your organization who partner with you to reach shared goals. You probably devote time and energy to nurturing partnership, knowing that healthy relationships don't happen by accident. If so, we applaud you and your hard work. We also know that you are devoting effort to building relationships in an atmosphere of multiple demands on you.

It's a New Day

It used to be that managers were not encouraged to cross turf lines. Sticking to your own staff and function and protecting them as your cherished turf have been valued approaches. Executives expected managers to stick to their knitting and do a good job of it. Managers focused on their own work, their own department, and their own team, letting other managers worry about theirs. They wanted their team to look good and sometimes kept others at a distance so they wouldn't be able to question what was really going on. Executives did not encourage managers to cross turf lines to solve system problems. Everyone had his or her responsibility and was supposed to take care of it.

Many of our systems and processes even supported internal competition rather than collaboration. Think about budget preparation, and how information and resources may or may not be shared. People fight for their piece of the pie, believing that "if I don't make demands, I won't get what I need." Competition became prevalent in the external environment as well, as leaders avoided sharing resources, equipment, and personnel. Everyone insisted upon doing it all, and alone, thinking little of the cost—or the customer.

These competitive ways won't serve us well in the future. The successful leader realizes the importance of building bridges with other leaders, of collaborating and creating partnership to achieve shared goals, partnership built on a foundation of mutual respect and trust.

Take a Look

How does turf protection look different from a relationship orientation in everyday life?

Fred

Fred is a new manager at Community Central. He finds that unavailability of wheelchairs has plagued Community Central for years. Because this touches so many departments, no one manager has been able to solve the problem—and recently, no one has tried. As a turf-protecting manager, Fred does nothing about it. He thinks, *Why stick my neck out, when this problem seems to have gone on for years?* He also fears that a solution might entail having others look at how his department functions, leading to visibility he prefers to avoid. He figures he'll wait for someone else to do something about it.

If Fred were relationship-oriented and not concerned about protecting his turf, he would approach others to pursue ways they can partner to address this long-standing problem. He understands that not being able to get a wheelchair when a patient needs one is intolerable. It's a problem that needs to be tackled, regardless of who has to initiate action to relieve the problem. So he pulls peers together and, without finger pointing or blaming, makes a case for change.

Delia and Joanne

Delia has had a history of competition and mistrust with Joanne, another manager. Both have found ways to work around one another, and neither person feels she is the problem. The behavior of both managers is affecting others throughout the organization.

As a turf-protecting manager, Delia continues the stalemate. She rationalizes, "I don't have to like or work with everyone." She feels comfortable working around Joanne rather than with her. Conflict-avoiding, Delia feels anxious at the thought of any process she would have to go through to improve the relationship. Since neither manager sees herself as responsible for the friction in their relationship, both have a ready excuse and the other to blame.

As a relationship-oriented manager, Delia does not wait for Joanne to act first. It is not easy for her, but she prepares to talk with Joanne about the issues interfering with a positive work relationship. After preparing, she arranges a meeting in which she initiates a courageous conversation.

Delia takes the first steps to work through the issues with Joanne, all for the good of the team and results. She also makes sure she doesn't make matters worse by asking others to choose sides.

Paul and Denise

Paul's team and Denise's team do not work well together. They share a mutual history of backbiting and finger pointing. As managers they have tried numerous times to work things out, but each team feels that "those people don't understand what we do."

Paul and Denise, each turf-protecting and looking out for their own group, defend their people and try to protect them from attack and accusation. Wanting to feel that they are doing a good job, they become defensive. Also, because it's hard to get their folks to admit imperfection, they can't give an inch in any discussion meant to improve the situation.

In contrast, committed to building relationships, Paul and Denise try to change these negative dynamics by helping their people get to know the folks "on the other side." They orchestrate ways for them to learn about the work they all do, as well as ways to support each other. Paul and Denise also set an example of teamwork by making sure they speak positively about one another and the other's team. They find ways to bring their teams together to solve the interdepartmental problems that pit people against each other.

Paul and Denise also spend time getting their own houses in order. Teams that spend time developing their internal relationships generally work more effectively with other teams and groups. This work takes time, and Paul and Denise support these team-building activities, committed to the payoffs for everyone. They also have to use their experience as an example so that other managers with similar issues will come to feel comfortable taking these brave steps.

What Worries You?

Are you stuck in old habits of turf protection? If you've been prone to protecting your turf in the past instead of opening up and reaching out beyond your direct span of control, this shift to relationship building impels you to question your knee-jerk reaction and to make sure you are not continuing in a turf-protecting way. This is not easy, as these behaviors and expectations may have served you well for a long time.

Are you afraid to go against the grain? If your organization isn't demanding teamwork, managers who stick their necks out may be viewed with suspicion.

Do you fear rejection? There may be individuals who don't respond positively, even if you reach out to them. They may reject your peace offerings and insist that you and your teams are to blame for the problems in the system.

Are you concerned about the time involved in tending to relationships? Building relationships requires time and commitment. You can't wish people to be different. There are steps to go through and no short cuts. Is this a concern of yours?

Are you afraid you might not have what it takes? It takes work, and possibly a new approach, to develop a supportive, trusting relationship.

Are you fearful that you might open a can of worms in the process? Many leaders think it's easier to work around people than to go through the hassle of trying to change patterns of behavior. Some managers are afraid of making things worse. People say "let sleeping dogs lie," meaning "I really don't want to make change."

What Do You Stand to Gain?

When you shift from turf protection to relationship building, *you reduce your stress and have fewer problems to solve.* Why? Everyone is on the same page and committed to the same goals. Interpersonal conflicts, after all, are among the greatest dissatisfiers on the job.

People keep things in proportion. When you get to know and understand your partners, little things do not get blown out of proportion. They are dealt with on the spot, without a tremendous amount of extra work and energy.

You don't have to watch your back. People will be with you, not against you. If you don't have to watch your back constantly, you have more time and energy to watch what is really important.

People cut you some slack. When you have positive, trusting relationships, you do not have to watch what you say and do. People understand who you are and are less likely to misunderstand your words and actions. They are also more forgiving should you make a mistake. You do not have to walk on eggshells with people who like and care about you.

You can have a positive influence on others. You might inspire others to support teamwork and thus create a more harmonious work environment.

You and your team earn a positive reputation as bridge builders, as a positive force. When your relationships are effective with your staff, you encourage talented people to stay.

What Can You Do? How Can You Do It?

If you choose to work with colleagues to break down barriers and forge new relationships, you may find it challenging, because turf protection may have offered you a sense of safety and comfort. You may need to become hyperconscious of your protective instincts. You may need to catch yourself and short-circuit what may be habitually turf-protecting behavior.

To ease your way, we've chosen a few powerful strategies (Exhibit 8.1) that you can use to build strong relationships with people in other parts of your organization, outside, and within your own team.

Exhibit 8.1. Your Relationship-Building Toolkit.

Strategy one: Adjust your mind-set.

Strategy two: Establish a solid foundation for your relationships.

Strategy three: Make agreements.

Strategy four: Keep your relationships on track.

The first strategy helps you adopt a collaborative mind-set. It helps you discover what you personally stand to gain by taking the first step in building a relationship.

With the second strategy, we present tools you can use to establish a solid foundation for flourishing partnership with others. These include ways to help you learn more about people professionally and personally, whether they are within your team, in another department, or outside the organization.

The third strategy includes straightforward approaches to getting your cards on the table. You'll learn how to ask for what you want and need from your partners.

The fourth strategy includes tools you can use to troubleshoot your relationships and keep them on track, healthy, and constructive.

Strategy One: Adjust Your Mind-Set

Earlier, we described worries you may have about abandoning turf protection and embracing relationship building as a pivotal role. This first strategy helps you identify thoughts you have that encourage protecting your turf instead of reaching out and building a relationship with others.

Do you think that focusing on interpersonal relationships is not what leaders should be doing? Do you think that team friction is inevitable and something you just have to tolerate and accept? Many managers think so, but we don't agree. You have more important ways to spend your precious energy and time than absorbing the stress and unfair workload caused by a nonexistent or strained relationship. Relationship issues are often perplexing, but the issues create a ripple effect on customers, your colleagues, and your team. Left unattended, relationship issues deplete your energy and weaken your resolve to chase after ambitious goals.

What do you stand to gain from attending to relationships in a determined fashion? Use this tool to find out.

⚒ Tool: What's in This for Me?

Purpose. This tool helps you assess the toll that relationship problems take on your team's morale and effectiveness.

Method. Think about this past week. In the table below, list the times that you or your team members were caught in an uncomfortable situation as a result of lack of teamwork or understanding between people. Write down the result of that discord.

List also the outcomes that would have been different or better had the team relationship been harmonious and constructive.

What Would Have Been Different?

Situation	Result	What Would Have Been Different Had Relationships Been Strong?
Example: You weren't informed of a meeting.	You weren't able to provide needed input.	You could have saved the team time and energy, not to mention the hard feelings, that resulted from the confrontations that took place.

Are you surprised by the amount of time and energy actually spent on issues that could be prevented if teams and individuals worked more collaboratively? Managers report that nearly a third of their time and energy is spent recovering from team disconnect. Unfortunately, the sheer number of managers who find themselves depleted by relationship issues supports the belief some people hold that there is little a manager can do about it. This belief triggers a sense of helplessness and supports the status quo.

Hogwash, we say! We think there is a great deal you *can* do to change your current reality; we believe that you *must* do it. Many of the problems we have in health care are difficult to change or fix. Many are even out of our control. But the one thing that we can control is how we work with and treat each other. Making improvements here can dramatically enhance our effectiveness, value, and image.

We are saddened by the many wonderful employees we have known who left their jobs because of stressful relationships and a painful lack of teamwork. Employees resent petty backbiting, finger pointing, and organizational politics; they feel they can no longer be productive, content, or even physically healthy in what they see as a toxic environment. They jump ship to find an organization where people cooperate with, value, and support each other.

If you are party to a strained relationship (or no relationship at all) where you sorely need one, consider using the tools described here to help you break new ground and cultivate partnerships that make you more gratified and effective.

Do you need a mind-set adjustment? Take a look at three of the most prevalent thoughts and fears of managers related to relationships. Consider the extent to which you share these thoughts and fears. If you do, we suggest ways you can reframe how you think about them, so that your self-talk helps you build a relationship that produces results and allows you to work in harmony with your coworkers.

Fearful thought number one: "If I make an effort to build relationships, others might see me as touchy-feely, and I'll lose my credibility."

It's true that in some organizations people view attention to relationships as soft. Do you agree? Equally important, do you care? Do you think it's important or unimportant to spend time and energy building collaborative relationships? Are you convinced this will benefit you, your team, and your customers? If so, stop letting other people's thoughts and fears influence you; decide what you want to think and think it. Think through how you, in the privacy of your own mind, can counter what others regard as the prevailing wisdom but what you regard as the malarkey holding back your organization.

Instead of worrying that you might be disregarded as touchy-feely, think *I know I am behaving in a way that helps our customers and our organization.* It's the people who see relationship building as touchy feely who mouth off at colleagues, fly off the handle, and treat others with disdain and disregard. If creating workplace harmony and building solid business partnership gives you the reputation of being touchy-feely, then take pride in it.

Fearful thought number two: "If I try to build relationships, I won't be successful with everyone."

Ah, so true and inevitable. There are people who won't be collaborative no matter what you do. But so what? If you try and they don't respond, is it you who failed? As you know, in any relationship it takes two to tango. You can only do your part. If you do your part and the other person doesn't, you can always conclude that "I tried to break down the barriers. I took the high road. I can't take responsibility for the other person's reactions."

Fearful thought number three: "I'm uncomfortable with conflict."

Few people are comfortable with conflict, and most people hate it altogether. The question is, Can you be effective without ever engaging in it? Can you handle it even though you would rather avoid it? Will you fall apart, or become frightened or overwhelmed? Will you lose control? Probably not. Apprehension in anticipation of conflict tends to be *much* worse than the reality. In the face of conflict, we are likely to survive; if we handle the conflict well, we end up in a better place with our colleagues and ourselves because of it.

If you try to arrange your work life to be free of conflict, you miss opportunities for learning and for a breakthrough. Thinking of conflict you've had with others, we bet you can identify good results that came in the form of new understanding, easing of strain, new commitment, greater harmony, fairer distribution of work, and more.

Take a minute to try this now.

✖ Tool: Thinking Your Way Through Conflict

Purpose. This tool identifies thoughts that help you face conflict constructively.

Method. Think about a good relationship you have in which you and the other person engaged in a conflict at some point. Perhaps you had a misunderstanding or disagreement. If so:

- What was the conflict?
- How did you both experience it?
- How did you both share and resolve the conflict?
- What did you experience or learn as a result?
- What good results came from the conflict?

What thoughts helped you face this conflict, learn from it, and produce positive results? Do you think thoughts like these?

- The tensions I feel, these too shall pass.
- It's better to get feelings out than keep them inside, where they fester.
- Conflict is normal and natural.
- No risk, no gain.

Reminding yourself of times when you have survived and benefited from conflict in a work relationship is a great way to help you reframe thoughts that otherwise hold you back. The important lesson is that you have choices. You can decide to talk to yourself and think in ways that nudge you out of your silo and encourage you to initiate improvement in a relationship.

Strategy Two: Create a Solid Foundation for Your Relationships

We hope you're convinced that you have a lot to gain from enhancing your work relationships. You also have a fix on the thoughts that encourage you to do the hard things needed to build and maintain these relationships. Next, we'll launch into action. What can you do to build a strong relationship in the first place?

First of all, you know that a healthy relationship and partnership is the result of hard work. It rarely just *happens.* For a relationship to flourish, three things are needed: common goals, shared values, and mutual needs.

First, common goals. If you and I don't want compatible things, we aren't going to work well together. People get into a great deal of trouble once they discover that a partnership never had a chance, because the individuals involved didn't have the same vision or goals in mind.

The same is true of shared values. We may aim for the same goal but have opposing ideas about how to achieve it. If we can't agree on how we want to work, how we want to conduct our business, or how we want to treat people in the process, we will have difficulty supporting one another.

Gail worked with a medical director who was trying to start a school-based health program. This leader met with considerable resistance from school officials, until he stepped out of his authority role and focused on their shared goal: helping inner-city children have the very best access to health care, thus reducing sick days and health crises.

The medical director also realized that, although there were many issues about governance and financial risk to be ironed out, all parties shared values related to the work and how families and kids should be treated.

The final and more elusive criterion for a healthy relationship has to do with mutual needs. For a relationship to work, both parties must get something from the deal. Both parties have to believe the other partner has something that they want and need.

Creating this sense of win-win has giant importance. As leaders, we must take time to get to know our colleagues ideally at both a personal and professional level, so we can discover our common goals, shared values, and mutual needs.

Think about some of the many people you interact with often at work. How well do you know them? No doubt, you know and understand some more than others, and this helps you be responsive to the other person's needs.

✖️ Tool: Whom Do You Know? (Scott, 1997d)

Purpose. This tool helps you explore the thoughts and feelings you have about your colleagues and the effect these thoughts and feelings have on your relationship and their behavior.

Method. Think about two partners. The first should be one whom you respect and like. The second should be someone you either don't respect or don't like. Complete the following chart to differentiate your knowledge of these two people.

Two Colleagues in Contrast

	Colleague You Like	Colleague You Don't Like
What does this person like best about his or her work?		
What does this person like least about his or her work?		
What are this person's personal and professional goals? Where would this person like to be three years from now?		
What is this person doing to achieve these goals?		
What do you know about this person on a personal level (e.g., hobbies, interests, family)?		
What makes this person care about work? What makes the person want to be successful?		
What does this person think about you and your relationship with him or her?		
How could you or your team help this person achieve important goals?		

How did you do? Most of us realize we don't know much about the people we don't like much. Typically, we tend to avoid these individuals. But there is a great lesson here when it comes to teamwork. We can't improve a relationship unless we understand our colleagues, what makes them tick, what's important to them. There are many questions you can ask to learn more about your colleagues. Select some that particularly interest you, and arrange times to talk with both the people you considered just above. We promise improved understanding from simply asking them these questions to learn more about their goals and values.

Asking appreciative questions is crucial to getting to know your colleagues. Some people think that the information will just come out. It doesn't. When we conduct team-building sessions, we are constantly amazed that people who have worked together for years often have no knowledge or understanding of their colleagues' enthusiasms, interests, or goals.

Getting well acquainted on a personal level is important, but it's not the be-all and end-all. You also have to understand the work that colleagues do, so you can understand them better and also grasp how your own work fits with theirs. Gail was asked to develop a program designed to support new residents. Interviewing residents helped her become familiar with their perceptions of their work. Better yet, shadowing residents on a twenty-four- or thirty-six-hour rotation helped Gail understand much better their frustrations and needs. Asking questions may help you get a glimpse, but walking in your colleague's shoes extends your understanding tremendously.

✖ Tool: Walk in Each Other's Shoes

Purpose. This tool helps you gain insight into the roles, frustrations, and challenges of your colleagues in other departments and areas of your organization or system.

Method. List the four people with whom you need the best relationships if you are to be effective in your job.

Call each one. Ask permission to shadow this person in their job for a day. Explain that "your work and mine intersect. This makes our relationship very important. I think I could bring more to our relationship if I better understood your job—your responsibilities, frustrations, goals, and challenges. Would you be willing to let me shadow you for a day, so I can really understand your job?"

Afterward, consider ways you can share, appreciatively and respectfully, your learning with the person you shadowed. Propose a better way to work together, now that you know more about your colleague's resources, challenges, and functions.

Your colleague may be a bit nervous at the thought of your shadowing, but most people are also flattered and welcome the opportunity.

So far, we've shared ways you can get to know colleagues in other parts of your organization. What about the relationships you have with people on your team? Most leaders admit that these relationships are not what they need to be. Again, you can influence the quality of these relationships and the work outcomes that spring from them. The relationship-building leader understands how important it is to create healthy team relationships in which team members respect their coworkers and devote energy to strengthening team relationships. If you have harmonious and productive team relationships, your people are likely to work more collaboratively not only with one another but also with people in other departments and areas of your organization or system.

In Chapter Eleven, we share several exercises you can use to strengthen relationships within your team. Specifically, they help your staff understand and appreciate one another's talents, likes, and dislikes with an eye to building coworker relationships associated with job satisfaction. Try them; we think you'll like them. Don't forget the next step: teambuilding exercises require follow-up so the experience and ideas can become agreement and commitment.

Strategy Three: Make Agreements

Getting to know other people and understanding the work they do helps you establish a strong foundation for collegial relationship, but it stops short of producing focused results. When you are about to engage in a substantive work project with another person or group, it pays to devote time to reaching explicit agreement about the nature of the partnership that will lead to the results you want. Reaching explicit agreement requires attention, discussion, and design.

We love this next tool. It stems from our belief that, when planning a work project with a colleague, it helps to lay your cards on the table. This tool is surprisingly flexible. Managers have used it to strengthen customer-supplier relationships, to set up a new project with a coworker, and even to improve their relationship with a boss.

⚒ Tool: The Partnership Dialogue (Scott, 1995)

Purpose. Along with a partner or colleague, with this tool you can lay your cards on the table about what an effective partnership requires.

Method. Initiate the following dialogue with a partner or colleague with whom you need a strong working relationship in order to meet an important business challenge.

The Partnership Dialogue

Why should we partner?	How will each of us benefit from a strong partnership? How will it help other people? How will it help the organization? What's our real goal?
How could we work together?	What's the vision? What are the possibilities for this partnership? How can we collaborate and work together?
What do we need from each other?	What do we need from each other to make this vision a reality? What do you bring? What do I bring? What structures or resources will we need to support this effort?
What if . . . and *why not*?	What are the barriers and obstacles to our making this partnership work? How could we let each other down? What could go wrong?
So, *what* are the first steps?	What must we do to make the partnership work (i.e., agendas, tasks, and time lines)? What is most important? What will be easiest to accomplish?
How can we tell if we're on track?	What systems could we put in place to monitor how we're doing? How will we know when it's working and when we need to make course corrections?

This dialogue gives you common ground on which to build and strengthen your relationship and also approach the specific work you jointly need to accomplish.

The next tool helps you go even further. It helps you and your colleague be explicit and clear about otherwise fuzzy expectations that you hold of each other.

Picture this example. Nursing and Pharmacy folks do interdependent work and need a collaborative relationship. Nursing expects Pharmacy to deliver the right meds at the right time. Pharmacy expects Nursing to request stat orders only if there is a true emergency. It turns out that Pharmacy is repeatedly late with regular deliveries, because there are so many stat orders to fill. Because Nursing can't count on regular delivery, it makes most of the orders stat orders. The result: considerable mutual resentment arises, services to patients suffer, and relationships grow strained.

Using the next tool, Nursing and Pharmacy talk about their frustration with each other. They explain the actions on the part of the other that drive them nuts. The manager and perhaps other representatives of each department get together to articulate their team's needs. Finally, they hammer out an agreement. It spells out how they will meet each other's needs consistently, reducing the havoc they have been wreaking on each other.

✪ Tool: Interdepartmental Partnership Contract

Purpose. This tool improves communication and cooperation between departments.

Method. Meet with a manager from another department to discuss the value of working collaboratively.

You and the manager each work with your own staff to determine what they need and expect from one another to meet customers' needs. Form a partnership team with the other manager, several frontline employees from each area who know the key processes between the two departments, and yourself.

The partnership team meets to discuss and come to agreement on the critical issues between your two services. Crystallize these agreements into a written draft of a partnership contract, one addressing the items shown in the following list.

Interdepartmental Partnership Contract

1. Customer partner needs and requirements

2. Supplier partner commitments and standards

3. Conflict resolution plan

4. Potential areas for process improvement

5. Monitoring plan

Have members of the partnership team take the draft they have created back to their coworkers for review and suggestions.

Reconvene the partnership team to discuss and incorporate appropriate suggestions. Prepare a final contract, including dates for review and updates. Distribute the signed document to all employees with a need to know. Each manager sets up improvement teams as needed to improve work processes.

Members of the partnership team monitor the effectiveness of the contract terms in their own department and periodically reconvene the partnership team to refine commitments and ensure continuing success.

Does this sound laborious? It can be, especially during development. But it's only laborious if agreement and commitment have not been clear and thus created preventable strain in the relationship and preventable service problems for customers.

Now, let's say you have solid relationships going at work. Let's say you're respected for the support and cooperation you extend to your colleagues. You have a harmonious team. You deal directly with other people across functional lines and reach agreements that aid effective interdependence.

Do you know what's sometimes satisfying, sometimes maddening about relationships? You can't control them single-handedly. Their intensity dips and swings. The degree of contact among the parties ebbs and flows. Most of all, there are precipitating events (resignation, outsourcing decision, executive turnover, politics, board pressure, new rules and regulations, and much more) that throw a monkey wrench into the relationship without your even seeing it coming. Knowing that a relationship will inevitably hit rocks and squalls, how do you keep it smooth, flexible, functional, and productive?

Strategy Four: Keep Your Relationships on Track

Do you have a maintenance agreement on a home appliance? Does someone come to your house to check your heating system a couple of times a year? It's ironic that we pay people to "clear the air" with our HVAC systems, but this kind of attention to upkeep in a work relationship is relatively rare. What if we gave our regular relationships this kind of ongoing attention, asking whether the quality and output are what we want and need?

Here are techniques that serve the purpose of a relationship check. They help you check in on your relationships and tend to them as needed. If you take them for granted without constant tending, you can expect some degree of erosion and resulting frustration at work over time.

- *Personal check-in:* This applies to a relationship you have with another leader. When you meet, say, "I believe you and I need a very good relationship, and I want to be sure to do my part. How do you think we're doing? What is working in our relationship? And what isn't working for you? What can you, I, or we do to make our relationship more effective?"
- *Partnership check:* If you have a partnership agreement or contract with another department, work out a maintenance agreement. For instance, propose monthly or bimonthly meetings to review performance. Simply ask, "How are we doing? What's working, and what isn't? What can we do to improve?"
- *Liaison team:* The liaison team consists of a couple of representatives of two interdependent services or functions. They meet over lunch monthly to identify issues between the two services and follow up by troubleshooting with their respective teams. One hospital we know has these liaison teams: nursing and labs, nursing and radiology, marketing and the heart center, marketing and patient relations, home care and care management, and human resources and allied health managers.
- *With your staff:* At your team meetings, pose a warm-up question that takes the pulse of the group. For instance, ask "How would you rate our teamwork lately on a scale from one to five?" Or "How do you think others view our team lately?" The point is to unearth thoughts, feelings, and perceptions related to your team, so you can identify relationship issues needing attention. This is a sort of maintenance check on your team.

Now, what if you have a strained relationship with another individual and you find it affecting your work, your team, or your results? Here's a favorite tool Wendy uses when she or a colleague wants to heal a strained work relationship.

⚒ Tool: Let's Have Lunch

Purpose. This tool creates new possibilities for harmony and collaboration with a person with whom you currently have a strained relationship.

Method. Initiate a lunch with your colleague, saying, "I want a great relationship with you. I'm hoping you'll join me for lunch because I would like to get to know you better and also talk about ways we can strengthen our working relationship."

At lunch, ask questions like those in the list below, being sure to take a turn in answering if your colleague suggests it.

Let's-Have-Lunch Questions

- A little history first: How did you become involved in health care? What attracted you?
- For as long as you've been in health care, which job have you found most satisfying? What were the high points of that job?
- What have you found to be most frustrating in your jobs or your field?
- No doubt you have had several achievements during your career. Would you mind telling me about one you're particularly proud of? What was your specific role in it?
- What do you appreciate in your current job? What is satisfying?
- What do you see as your main challenges?
- Now, about our relationship and perceptions of each other:

  From your perspective, what do you see as my strengths? What do you appreciate about me?

  What do I do that frustrates you? Please tell me what I do and what you see as the consequences.

  What do you wish I would do to make our relationship better?
- Now, about this conversation:

  Any surprises?

  Given our goal of having a productive, mutually respectful relationship, what working agreements do you think would help us stay on track?

How might we check in with each other to discuss how we're doing?

- Gracious thanks!

You'll be amazed at the fruits of this caring conversation. The knowledge and respect you communicate to each other is like money in the bank when and if your relationship becomes stressed.

What do you do when you find yourself upset, annoyed, or frustrated with a colleague's behavior, and it's too late to start from scratch in building the relationship? In this situation, you need skill in giving respectful, constructive, and timely feedback to the person. This next tool is an effective structure for giving feedback to a colleague in hopes of fixing the problem while also strengthening, not harming, your relationship.

⚒ Tool: Feedback Model

Purpose. This tool delivers constructive feedback while helping you preserve a healthy, respectful relationship.

Method. Plan your feedback ahead of time, so you can word it well and make it optimally effective. Use the following language model, and you'll get the best results.

Model for Great Feedback

Describe:	Helpful Words	An Example
Your positive intention	"I am talking to you because I want a really good relationship with you."	I want a great relationship with you and want to share some feedback with you. OK?
The situation	"The situation is . . ."	I need to turn in the financial report by this afternoon. You agreed to provide me with the statistics by yesterday afternoon.
The problematic behavior that did or didn't happen	"As I see it, you . . ."	You didn't provide it, and you didn't call to let me know the problem.

Describe:	Helpful Words	An Example
The consequences for you, your team, customers, the organization	"The consequences are . . ."	I'm going to be late turning in the report, and my boss is going to give me a hard time about it.
A pinch of empathy	"Now, I realize that you might have . . ."	Now, I realize things can come up that you didn't anticipate—things that interfere with your putting together the information for me.
Your hope or expectation	"In the future, I'm hoping you will . . ."	In the future, I hope you'll do all you can to meet a deadline you commit to. If you can't, let me know in time for me to get what I need another way."

If you withhold feedback, you miss an opportunity to make your relationship better. With this model, you'll be able to say everything you want to say respectfully.

Last but not least, to keep your relationships on course, we want to share a few tips, this time in the form of what *not* to do if you want to sustain healthy work relationships (Exhibit 8.2).

An Investment with a Welcome, Stress-Reducing Return

As you undoubtedly know from your personal life, relationships take careful tending. The same is true for work relationships. Yet at work, there is the danger of being so focused on tasks and getting the work done that you take relationships for granted. That's when they fall apart, making your work much harder and results much more difficult to achieve.

Consider relationships as a phenomenally rich resource you have at your disposal. By establishing and sustaining healthy relationships at work, you trigger a multiplier effect. You release energy and productivity. You produce results that

Exhibit 8.2. Relationship Killers.

1. Going around your colleagues instead of dealing with them directly
2. Making promises and then proceeding to break them
3. Coming late to meetings, indicating disrespect for others' time and an exaggerated view of the importance of yours
4. Turning your staff against each other: making insinuating comments or undermining remarks to staff, so that they join you in feeling animosity toward a colleague
5. Expecting your colleague to read your mind, instead of saying what you want or need
6. Doing a halfhearted or sloppy job when you commit to doing something for this person
7. Wasting the person's time at meetings by not preparing
8. Taking up your colleague's time, while disregarding cues that suggest "not now"
9. Expecting your colleague to support your needs, but holding back your support
10. Not returning phone calls, communicating that your colleague is unimportant
11. Treating your colleague with disrespect, calling it a "style thing" on your part, and expecting the person to adjust to your style
12. Getting defensive when you receive feedback
13. Complaining about your colleague to higher-ups, before you've done all you can possibly do to deal with the person directly

come only through collaboration. You help to create a positive, nurturing work climate. You are a role model for your staff. Your healthy relationships have a dynamo effect on recruitment and retention.

You are not soft-minded when you step out of your silo and nurture effective relationships with others. You are a manager who recognizes the pivotal role that relationships play in your job effectiveness and who has the courage, ambition, and vision to build bridges for the sake of your own peace of mind, your effectiveness, your team, and your value to your organization.

9

From Function Manager to Business Leader

For years, health care organizations have been organized along functional lines. The structure supported a system in which managers defined their main job as focusing on internal operations and keeping their department running smoothly. Although smooth functioning has certainly benefited customers and the organization, these days managers need to take on broader responsibility, running their services like businesses that they own, businesses that they want to grow, to make lean and mean, to strengthen, to make distinctive and impressive in the eyes of customers.

A Revealing Look in the Mirror

True or False?	True	False
1. I spend most of my time focusing on internal operations.	____	____
2. When I devote time to learning, I tend to focus on learning what is state-of-the-art in my field.	____	____
3. When there is a downturn in business, I cut expenses.	____	____
4. When systems are working, I leave well enough alone.	____	____
5. I seem to jump from one crisis to another all day long.	____	____
6. I focus on making sure my department meets requirements.	____	____
7. In the last month, I have learned about other organizations' best practices in my field.	____	____
8. I spend some time every week in direct contact with customers.	____	____
9. I spend some time every week doing strategic things.	____	____
10. I have implemented new business ideas within the last month.	____	____

If you considered the first five statements false and the last five true, you have made the shift from functional manager to business leader. But what exactly does this mean?

A person with the mind-set of a functional leader thinks, *My main goal in my job is to keep things running smoothly.* A business leader considers this essential to doing a good job, but it does not alone constitute success. The business leader wants to go beyond smooth operation to add value in other ways: staying in close touch with customers, growing the business, outdoing a competitor, improving customer service, reducing unnecessary expense, pursuing a new business opportunity, and most likely *all* of these. Business leaders see themselves as strategists. They don't leave this to executives.

In the face of financial difficulties, the business leader looks not only for ways to reduce cost but also for ways to generate additional revenue. When a business leader has an innovation or improvement in mind, he or she does considerable homework to evaluate its potential and, when convinced of its value, advances it relentlessly.

People with a business leader mind-set make a concerted effort to understand the big picture. They lead their function or service with a sense of ownership and entrepreneurial zeal. The functional manager's focus is largely inside out (on systems, methods, policies, teams); the focus of the business leader is more often outside in (on customers and their needs, the marketplace, the competition, and emerging trends that affect the business).

Also, they steward the organization's resources as if they were their own. They take initiative and spearhead innovation and improvement. They seek to keep things going and keep the business growing. They think like owners: *If it is to be, it's up to me.*

It's a New Day

In today's complex and demanding health care world, with so many lines of business and so many functions that must support the lines of business, a health care organization needs every manager to be a business leader. Senior executives used to handle the strategic thinking for the organization and rarely engaged middle managers in the process. Competitive pressures today overburden senior executives with too much to figure out. They need us at the middle management level to step up to the plate and engage in strategic thinking and planning. We must run our piece of the action, and manage the interdependencies with other parts of the organization and our market so that services are seamless, growth plans constructive, and business relationships solid.

With such hefty demands on the health care leader, every manager has to share responsibility for the overall business goals. Functional management is limited. It's constrained—with walls around it. This stands in the way of partnership and creative linkage that lead to important positive outcomes.

Take a Look

Here's how functional management looks different from business leadership in everyday situations.

Mel

Mel is the new director of food services at Memorial Hospital. Memorial administrators respected the former director, and people are telling Mel that Food Services operated fine in the past. Initially, it looks that way to him too. Now, after taking some time to learn about how the department works and who does what, he realizes that he could run the department better and at lower cost if he were to redesign certain processes and rearrange certain people's schedules.

If Mel sees himself as a functional manager, he may not initiate these changes: "This department has been respected. Why fix what isn't broken?" He flows with the tide until such time as the hospital's finances press administrators to ask managers, including Mel, to offer up cuts.

Thinking as a business leader, he sees this situation differently: "This is a waste of precious resources." He proceeds with service redesign to free up staff resources and employ the freed-up people and hours to enhance Food Services in a way that benefits the patient. He is not comfortable consuming resources unnecessarily or inefficiently, since this reduces the dollars he has at his disposal to provide excellent food and services.

Laura

The cost of pharmaceuticals in Community Hospital's employee benefits plan is growing astronomically, in keeping with the national trend. At the half-year point, pharmacy benefit expense at Community shows a variance above budget in excess of a million dollars. At a meeting of hospital pharmacists, Laura, who directs Community's pharmacy department, hears about a nearby hospital that opened an in-house pharmacy for its own employees. Apparently, the in-house pharmacy in its first year had controlled this hospital's cost and also improved convenience for employees. Intrigued, Laura runs the idea past her boss, who responds: "Sounds complicated. I'm not sure we have the space for it, and I'm not sure we could save money by the time we hire people to run it."

Thinking as a functional manager, Laura knows that her boss isn't hot on the idea, but "I'll leave well enough alone and let Human Resources worry about reducing pharmacy benefit expenses."

Thinking as a business leader, Laura takes a closer look at what has the potential to be a great opportunity to enhance services to employees, while reducing soaring benefit costs. Although she knows this project could mean a gargantuan amount of work, she looks into it further and arranges to visit the colleague who instituted the in-house pharmacy. After learning much more about it, she roughs out a business plan that describes the goals and approach and estimates its return on investment (ROI). She then takes this plan and the ROI figures to her boss and advocates for it assertively. Laura approaches the project as an entrepreneur approaches a new business opportunity: with determination and zeal.

Hal

Hal runs a clinical service for Hudson Hospital. Because he has been preoccupied with staff turnover and arrival of new equipment, he has not paid much attention to the first few months' financial reports for his service.

Hal receives a current report and thinks he'd better take a good look at how his service is doing. Exhibit 9.1 shows an important piece of the report.

Whether Hal thinks like a functional manager or a business leader, he is likely to draw these conclusions from the data:

- Expenses are below budget. This is good.

- But volumes are less than those budgeted. This isn't good.

- The resulting cost per unit is higher than budgeted, creating a bottom-line problem.

Seeing himself as a functional manager, Hal feels good that actual expenses are lower than budgeted expenses and concludes that he has been controlling expenses well, even though volume expectations are below budget. He thinks he might have to cut expenses even further to bring the cost per unit in line with the budget.

Exhibit 9.1. Hal's Monthly Report.

Volume Variance			Expense Variance			Cost per Unit		
	Month-to-date	Year-to-date		Month-to-date	Year-to-date		Month-to-date	Year-to-date
Actual volume	624	3,399	Actual expense	$277,420	$1,400,701	Actual cost per unit	$444	$412
Budgeted volume	666	3,531	Budgeted expense	$284,693	$1,449,315	Budgeted cost per unit	$427	$410
Variance	(42)	(132)	Variance	($7,273)	($48,614)	Variance	$17	$2

Note: () indicates under budget.

Thinking as a business leader, he homes in on the fact that volume is falling below budget, bringing the cost per unit up to the point of producing a shortfall. He calls people together to inquire, "Why the decline in volume?" Then he schemes about how he and others can build this volume within a short time frame. He may develop a list of business prospects he hasn't talked with in a while and schedule himself for networking visits that he hopes to convert into referrals.

His head does not go immediately to cost cutting, but rather to how he can build the business.

In these cases, both the functional manager and the business leader may appear effective. However, the business leader tackles problems aggressively, takes responsibility for cultivating business, and delivers better overall results.

What Worries You?

With the complexity of systems, people, and customer needs functional managers have had to manage and address, this can be a difficult transition—hard, time-consuming, and a bit scary.

Are you worried about finding time to manage operations and do strategic thinking? Taking on a strategic role does require you to rise above the fray of everyday operations and get the view from thirty thousand feet. Protecting time for strategic thinking while juggling operational responsibility certainly does require some extraordinary self-discipline.

If you're living in a paternalistic culture, are you concerned that your opinions, decisions, and plans don't really matter? Although in some cultures a manager who acts like a business leader may not get the support needed to bring plans to fruition, if you don't act like a business leader you're likely to have no chance at all.

Are you concerned that you don't have access to complete information? Taking on responsibility to make far-reaching decisions about your business, you will be relying on the information available to you.

Are you afraid to chase after ambitious goals? Some managers perceive this as frightening, overwhelming, or unmanageable, given other responsibilities and priorities in their lives.

Do you find accountability anxiety-provoking and seek to avoid it? Overall, the functional manager is likely to feel safer, more comfortably competent, and more in control than the business leader.

Are you worried that you cannot learn the hard-nosed skills a business leader needs? Business leadership does require knowledge of business skills, such as marketing, finance, accounting, operations management, and much more. If you have not been trained in business skills or if you have not had experience as a generalist and been exposed to these skills on the job, the need to learn these skills may create new pressure to learn new skills—on top of those you already face in your demanding job.

What Do You Stand to Gain?

These worries stop some managers from pursuing the shift to business leadership, but making the shift produces overriding benefits:

- *Business leaders feel challenged, never bored.* When you assume the role of business leader, you have a *big and complicated* job to do. This may be energizing to you, bringing you engagement and welcome challenges.

- *With added accountability, you can take pride in your results.* Many managers feel vital when they are responsible for producing visible results. They enjoy a sense of accomplishment.

- *You intermingle with people in all parts of your organization.* If you enjoy diverse relationships and the cross-fertilization that comes from working with other people in other fields, you may find business leadership much more gratifying than functional management. Business leaders recognize the limits of their control too, but they do not let this stop them. They initiate interdepartmental initiatives and problem solving, so that they can try to affect the forces beyond their area that could be helping (or may be hurting) their service's effectiveness.

- *You gain the respect of customers and your organization's executives.* Because of your determined efforts to develop the business, meet customer expectations, and deliver positive results, others admire you.

- *You have opportunities to learn and grow.* As new market challenges present themselves and you compel yourself to respond effectively, you inevitably engage in learning.

- *You make things happen.* With your competitive instincts sparked, your resourcefulness, and your responsibility for the whole of your business, you can get things done, improve outcomes, and find solutions to longstanding problems . . . in short, get results.

What Can You Do? How Can You Do It?

If you choose to move in the direction of business leadership, here are five core strategies to help you grow yourself (Exhibit 9.2).

Exhibit 9.2. Your Business Leader's Toolkit.

Strategy one: Think like a business leader—with a sense that you own the business.

Strategy two: Act strategically.

Strategy three: Use business acumen to advance your proposals and initiatives.

Strategy four: Use resources effectively.

Strategy five: Take responsibility for results and course corrections.

The first strategy helps you think like a business owner, because thinking this way pushes you to set priorities and act like a business leader in your daily activities.

The second strategy helps you embrace the importance of acting strategically. When you think like an owner, you are responsible for the fate of the business. If you don't think strategically about it, your business will wallow in the status quo.

Strategy number three helps you develop business acumen and use it when you want to advance a proposal or idea. The tools here help you do important homework and then sell your proposals effectively.

The fourth is very important to most administrators; it is about efficient, effective use of resources. With the plaguing resource constraints that are an everyday fact of life, you stretch the available dollars and also gain considerable respect by becoming a skillful planner and conserver of resources.

Strategy number five supports you in taking responsibility for results and tracking these results so as to make timely course corrections.

We want to mention also that the tools in Chapter Seven ("From Busyness to Results") are a great addition to the business leader's toolkit presented in this chapter.

Strategy One: Think Like a Business Leader, with a Sense That You *Own* the Business

Business leaders treat their domain as their own business, believing that they can indeed make the business unit successful. There are certainly limits to this in a big organization, but people who think like a business leader act in ways that contribute optimally to the organization's mission and bottom line.

Dare we say that the mental model that tends to drive the functional manager role is paternalistic? The parents (the executives) drive the entire process, taking responsibility for the overall business, strategic planning, divvying up jobs, and monitoring to make sure people are doing them. A business owner's mental model for this aspect of their role is more likely that of an autonomous adult with authority, responsibility, and accountability.

How does a business owner think? Find out more by using the next tool to interview a business owner you know.

⚒ Tool: The Business Leader's Innermost Thoughts

Purpose. This tool helps you understand the thought patterns of a business leader, so you can entertain these thoughts yourself.

Method. Identify a successful business leader or someone you think demonstrates the characteristics of one in your organization. Schedule and conduct an interview with this person using the approach in Exhibit 9.3. Take notes of key words and thoughts, so you can refer to them later.

Afterward, sort through your notes and write down the essence of this business leader's thinking. Ask yourself which of those thoughts you have. Which ones would you like to think more often?

Finally, reprogram yourself. Write down your preferred thoughts, one per note card, and flip a card face up on your desk daily.

If you enjoy this interview, pick other inspirational business leaders you know and interview them too. The more exposure you give yourself to the mental maps of business leaders, the more you will think as they do, using your own self-talk to bolster your effectiveness.

Exhibit 9.3. The Thinking of a Business Leader: Interview.

Introduction

I'm interested in learning more about how an effective business leader thinks. I view you as an effective business leader and would like to ask you a few questions. OK?

Questions

1. What is an example of an accomplishment you've had in your role as business leader that you feel proud of?

2. I'm trying to understand how a business leader thinks—you in particular. When you were first approaching the experience you just described, what thoughts ran through your head? (Push for more and more.)

3. What is an example of a time when you felt your business was taking a downturn? In that case, what thoughts ran through your head?

4. If you were teaching a class of managers to become business leaders and wanted to tell them the thoughts that characterize business leaders, what thoughts would you describe?

   Your thoughts about higher-ups when you need their permission to move forward on a plan

   Your thoughts about failure

   Your thoughts about growth and building business

   Your thoughts about your team

   Your thoughts when you face obstacles

   Your criteria for success

   Your thoughts about yourself

5. While I have you here, let me ask you also: What are the critical skills a manager needs to become a business leader?

6. (If person knows you) You know me. I want to perform as a business leader. What advice can you give me to help me achieve that?

Closing

Thanks! I admire your approach to your work, and I also greatly appreciate your sharing your thoughts, experiences, and advice with me.

Going further with thinking like a business leader, functional managers see themselves as wearing *many* hats; business leaders wear *different* hats. In this next tool, take a look at yourself to identify which hats of the business leader you already wear and which you think you need to build into your wardrobe.

⚒ Tool: Snapshot of Your Role

Purpose. This tool helps you identify those roles of the business leader that you currently assume (as opposed to having to learn to assume).

Method. Which of the critical roles in Exhibit 9.4 do you think are important to your job? Check off those that are.

Think of and jot down a recent example of when you played one of these important roles. Finally, identify any roles that, on second thought, you could stand to incorporate into your vision of your role.

The point: you need to see your role as one of business leader, with these rich and diverse subparts that make up total responsibility—ownership—for a business unit and its performance. Does it sound as though you need to do it all? You do, but with help. Find out how other managers do this. Draw them into your deliberations. Stretch your capabilities by taking on a role that you have not previously played, and you will bring great value to your organization.

One other critical piece of the thinking process of the business leader has to do with external versus internal orientation.

The functional manager tends to engage in inside-out thinking. How do we do things? What are the effects on patients and other customers? In contrast, the business leader engages in outside-in thinking, attending to what's happening in the industry and among competitors, and considering the forces in the outside world that have an effect inside.

Effective businesspeople seek to understand their competitors' strengths, weaknesses, and strategies. They are market-driven. They know who their customers are and how these customers make decisions. They take pains to stay in tune with their customers' needs and concerns, and they strategize and regroup to meet customer needs better than their competitors do.

Exhibit 9.4. A Snapshot of Your Role.

Critical Roles	Important to My Job	Example for Food Services Department	I Need to Incorporate
Responsible for aligning business unit with mission and goals of organization		New "your choice" menu helps meet individual needs critical to patient satisfaction	
Responsible for staff understanding of how they fit into the big picture		Engage staff in dialogue on their role in patient satisfaction	
Responsible for revenue, not cost control alone		Reconsider pricing strategy; introduce catering services	
Decision maker		Decision to expand cafeteria hours; decision to start coffee kiosks	
Strategic planner; responsible for strategy		Visit other organizations for best practices; discuss vision with key stakeholders	
Marketing strategist; direct dealing with marketplace to generate opportunity		Offer catering services to community groups; start community health newsletter; dietitian-run weight loss support groups	
Relationship building with customers and actual or potential partners; networker		Figure out optimal services with new merger partner; contact other facility about locating coffee kiosks there; meet with long-term care facility about needed improvements	
Resource hunter		Find lower-cost, higher-quality vendors	
Process designer		Reconfigure food stations to improve traffic flow	
Troubleshooter; oil the wheels and remove barriers		Work with loading dock on on-time deliveries; make strong case for more efficient, higher-capacity dishwasher	
Evaluator; track results		Implement success indicators for coffee kiosks; survey patients and nurses on new "your choice" menus	
Responsible for actively learning and making course corrections		Train dietitians and nurses on "your choice" menu system; in-service for hostesses; in-service for chefs on catering services	

The next tool helps you take a look at the extent to which you are an outside-in thinker in your approach to your job.

✖ Tool: Outside-In Thinking

Purpose. This tool helps you pinpoint the extent to which you are an outside-in thinker.

Method. In the privacy of your office, ask yourself how much of the information in Exhibit 9.5 you know and have made known to your team and boss. The extent to which you and your colleagues know these things indicates your degree of engagement in the kind of outside-in thinking characteristic of the business leader.

If you see lots of checks in Exhibit 9.5, you are already engaged in outside-in thinking. If you don't, the blank boxes point you to the need to pursue environmental scanning and learning opportunities, to help you shift your thinking from inside-out to outside-in.

That's all about how you think and how you perceive your role. Assuming your thoughts now align with business leadership, let's look at a select few skills and processes that are vital to it, starting with the skills involved in acting strategically.

Strategy Two: Act Strategically

Health care managers who engage in the role of business leader apply tried-and-true business practices to their work. Rather than devoting all of their time to what can be the consuming and endless quagmire of everyday operational challenges, they dedicate prime time to strategic activity:

- They scan the environment to learn about trends, competitors, customers, partners, threats, and opportunities outside their business.

- They recognize the broad implications of trends and issues and apply them to forming strategy.

- They identify strategic opportunities and capitalize on them.

- They develop strategic alliances.

- They make strategic twists and turns in response to changing conditions and opportunities.

Exhibit 9.5. Outside-In Thinking.

	I'm Quite Aware of This	I've Made My Boss Aware of This	I've Made My Team Aware of This
What national trends present new challenges and opportunities for our organization and my team's work?			
What state trends present new challenges and opportunities for our organization and my team's work?			
What local trends present new challenges and opportunities for our organization and my team's work?			
What is happening in our organization's immediate community or primary service area that presents new challenges and opportunities to our organization and my team's work?			
Who are our customers, and what are their demographics?			
What do our customers want and expect?			
What trends are likely to shape their wants and expectations in the future?			
Who are our main competitors?			

Exhibit 9.5. (continued)

	I'm Quite Aware of This	I've Made My Boss Aware of This	I've Made My Team Aware of This
What are our competitors' strengths?			
What are our competitors' weaknesses?			
What are our competitors' main competitive strategies?			
What regulations are in the works?			
What technology advances are in the works that affect my team?			
What educational opportunities are out there to upgrade our effectiveness?			
What quality standards are the norm and the leader in our industry?			
How can we favorably differentiate or position ourselves from our competitors?			

This first tool for acting strategically offers you a format for profiling your business and business strategy comprehensively. Business leaders think through their mission, the vision of the business, the values by which they want to operate, strategies pivotal to reaching their goals, and how to track performance. They engage in planning to get a total picture of where they are going and how to get there. And they do this for themselves, their boss, and their team. This kind of plan helps them build and sustain momentum.

⚙ Tool: My Business Profile

Purposes. This tool allows you to describe your business unit and its mission, goals, and strategies in a nutshell; it helps you develop a roadmap for your services.

Method. Take a crack at filling out the chart in Exhibit 9.6.

If you can complete this chart, you are already taking responsibility for mapping your business goals and strategy. If not, consider going through a process with your team in which you develop this profile to guide your work in the coming year.

The next tool, the balanced scorecard, is all the rage—and for good reason. It helps you maintain focus and balance. As a business leader, you may find yourself plagued by competing priorities and pressures. You have to meet the changing expectations of your various customer groups. You have multiple goals, relating to care delivery, research, growth, effective resource use, education, and the like.

The balanced scorecard (Kaplan and Norton, 1996) is a wonderful framework that helps you identify a balanced set of key measures that you then use to drive your strategies, monitor results, and communicate with your various constituencies about your priorities.

⚙ Tool: Focusing with the Balanced Scorecard

Purpose. This tool is a framework for developing a balanced scorecard for your business unit.

Method. The balanced scorecard has two key components. The first, the strategy map, is a visual representation of your overall strategy. It helps you organize your strategic objectives with four perspectives in mind:

Exhibit 9.6. My Business Unit in a Nutshell.

Mission of overall organization					
Mission of my business unit; how it contributes to the overall mission					
My business unit's key customers (internal or external) and their main needs					
Our main products or services					
Our niche or distinction that provides unique value to our customers					
Vision for how this business unit will serve this purpose					
Key values: *how* team will operate in pursuit of mission, in the service of our customers					
Our top three strategic initiatives for this year	What?	Goals (e.g., volume, bottom line, revenue)	Time frame	How we'll evaluate	Who's responsible
1.					
2.					
3.					
Resource needs					
How we'll evaluate our success: milestones and yardsticks					

financial, customer, internal processes, and learning. By articulating your strategy from all four perspectives, you achieve balance. You reduce the risk of your strategy being driven too much by one perspective or another.

Yardsticks are the second component. This part involves a mix of performance indicators that enable you to see how you're doing and to make timely course corrections.

With these in place, you are in a much better position to set strategic priorities and allocate resources in line with these priorities.

The diagram below shows a framework for a strategy map for an emergency department.

Emergency Department Strategy Map

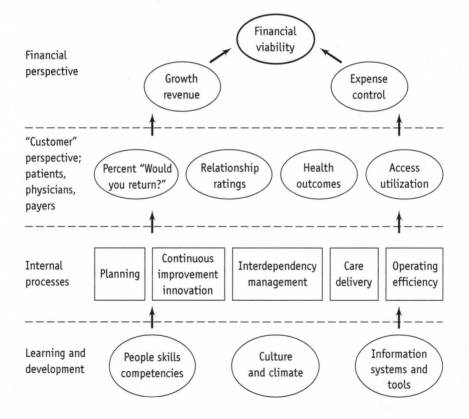

Note: Modeled after Strategy Map in "Implement the Balanced Scorecard . . ." (1996).

Associated with each box or oval, you develop a yardstick or measuring device so that you can monitor performance over time from all perspectives.

Create a roadmap for your service. Work with your team to develop it. You might have an implicit roadmap that you think people understand, but the process of making this explicit usually uncovers the reality that people may not be on the same page.

Perhaps you are thinking, *Map or no map, how will I ever have time for strategy?* Consider this next tool, which we view as a magic carpet that transports you in the face of seemingly endless demands into a strategic zone. The strategic sabbatical is based on the truism that it's hard to be operational and strategic at the same time.

⊗ Tool: The Strategic Sabbatical

Purpose. This tool helps you discipline yourself to think strategically.

Method. Devote one full day a month to strategic thinking. Create a one-day haven for yourself in which you let go of operational pressures and dream up possibilities. Spend this day off site, or exploring the Web, or making a best-practice visit, or reading, or talking to a colleague in another organization, or going to a seminar, or having a freewheeling discussion with a member of your team.

At the end of the day, write down your gleanings and share them with your colleagues.

Consider this activity for your coworkers too. It gets people to kick around strategies and opportunities in a constant swirl of creative possibility, fueled by stimulation from the vast world outside your organizational walls.

Even if you embrace the need to engage in strategic thinking in your role as business leader, this is nothing more than rhetoric unless you make the time to do it. The great news is that the payoff is amazing. We guarantee it.

Strategy Three: Use Business Acumen to Advance Your Proposals and Initiatives

Let's say you've done strategic thinking and identified an opportunity for process improvement, business growth, or improved patient satisfaction. The next tool helps you apply business acumen to advocate for and advance your proposal, moving the initiative from fantasy to reality.

People who are successful in business engage in thorough research, analysis, and planning before they implement even the brightest of their ideas. Simply put, they do their homework, so they can determine if their idea is likely to produce the desired benefits.

Do you know how to perform a return-on-investment analysis when you have an idea, service, or project you want to pursue? This next tool offers a simple approach.

⚙ Tool: A Straightforward Approach to ROI

Purpose. This tool can be used to analyze the return on investment of your ideas, to build confidence in these ideas for yourself and others.

Method. Use the worksheet in Exhibit 9.7 as a template for a basic ROI analysis.

Present your proposal in an organized fashion using this same outline. Higher-ups will respect your depth of information and be more likely to give you the go-ahead, since they can see you have left no stone unturned.

Remember that business leaders feel the money they are spending is from their own pocket even when it isn't. They take the question "Is it worth it?" very, very seriously. Embedded in the ROI analysis is scrutiny of the return on the plan you're proposing. In some situations, a full-fledged ROI analysis may not be appropriate, but great care about resource use is still critical.

Strategy Four: Use Resources Effectively

In everyday decisions and in response to emerging problems and needs, business leaders are conscious of how they use resources, even more so when they find they have not anticipated and budgeted the expense.

Exhibit 9.7. A Homegrown Approach to an ROI.

The opportunity you recognize:

The essence of your proposal: "What I/we propose is . . ."

Who is in on this proposal with you, and why?

The need or rationale: Why is it important to do this?

Who are your customers? What are the main benefits, payoffs, or positive results you can expect for these customers and stakeholders?

- Patients, families, community
- Doctors
- Employees
- The organization
- The decision maker(s)

Revenue implications: How much? Over what period of time? Years one, two, three?

The price tag and costs involved (whether to generate the level of revenue projected or provide the services or benefits described):

The risks involved and barriers to success (including likely resistance to this proposal): Right off the bat, what are the "yes, buts" and "what ifs"?

Your concrete plan, with time line:

What you need up-front and down the line to make it happen (e.g., approval, collaboration, guidance, operating funds, capital investment in equipment, time, etc.):

ROI (the punch line)—the return on investment (whether revenue or not, how and why potential benefits outweigh costs and risks):

The consequences of not going forward with this:

In the face of customer and staff frustration, some managers immediately want to throw money and more staff at the problem. That may solve some problems and apply to investing in some opportunities, but you only know this if you first look for ways to avoid adding expense. If you have a business leader mind-set in the face of problems, you first look for process improvement that can ease the problem. In the face of an opportunity, you first look at how you can, with existing resources, pursue it. Because of today's maddening financial constraints, we all need to excel at effective resource use, working from a sense that we share responsibility for making ends meet.

This next tool helps you ask critical questions as you face a problem or opportunity that appears to require additional resources.

✪ Tool: Trigger Questions on Effective Use of Resources

Purpose. This tool guides your thinking so that you use resources efficiently and effectively, avoiding unnecessary expense.

Method. Keep these questions handy and ask them the next time you face a problem or opportunity that appears to require additional funds or staff:

- Assuming no more money, how can we still do what we want to do? What's a creative way to do it that doesn't require so many resources?

- Assuming we cannot hire more staff to do this, how can we shift the work of existing staff, or partner with others so that we can free up staff time for this without having to pay more for it?

- Assuming we can shift money from one place to another within our scope, how can we free up funds for this?

- Can we make our current work processes more efficient, freeing up resources for this plan?

- If we have to get approval to spend money on this plan, what offset can we offer up to our higher-ups, so that we keep our services budget neutral?

Engage your staff and colleagues in other departments to help you consider these questions. People piggyback on one another's ideas and achieve better ideas as a result of group synergy.

Thinking like an owner, ROI analysis, strategic thinking, effective resource use—all of these help you demonstrate the kind of business acumen your organization needs from you, given its multiple priorities, tough business challenges, and increasingly complex world.

Business Leaders Are Respected Contributors

Have you heard this? There are three kinds of managers: those who make things happen, those who watch things happen, and those who wonder what happened. Health care managers with a business leader mind-set do not rely on instructions or directives from above. They do not wait to be asked to take initiative. Business leaders make things happen proactively, responsibly, strategically, and accountably, producing great results for their customers, the organization, and their own track record and marketability.

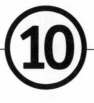

From Employee-as-Expendable to Employee-as-Precious

Employees quit their managers more often than they quit their jobs. The old-school belief—that "they should be lucky to have a job"—reflects a blind spot about the importance of employees to your services. Perceiving your team members as *individuals* worthy of respect and care, and also as your organization's most precious resources, is pivotal to retaining talented people, and, through them, attracting even more.

A Revealing Look in the Mirror

True or False?	True	False
1. I don't know enough about my staff members to be able to inquire about their lives outside of work in a caring way.	_____	_____
2. The needs of the organization drive my decisions about staff work schedules.	_____	_____
3. Because all jobs have their frustrations, I don't go to great lengths when my staff complain about obstacles that they say make their jobs difficult.	_____	_____
4. I think people should keep their personal issues out of the workplace.	_____	_____
5. In the event of a conflict between an employee's family and work responsibilities, I am very annoyed when the job suffers.	_____	_____
6. When a new staff member comes on board, I provide a really terrific welcome and orientation.	_____	_____
7. When staff members express concerns, I take their concerns very seriously and make sure I respond in a timely fashion.	_____	_____
8. I try to remove barriers and obstacles, so my staff can be successful.	_____	_____
9. I do specific things to build identification with our team, because I want my staff to feel connected to one another.	_____	_____
10. When an individual on my staff wants special arrangements to make the job more doable, I try hard to accommodate the person's needs.	_____	_____

If you answered false to the first five items on the quiz and true to the last five items, you don't consider employees to be expendable or replaceable. To the contrary, you appreciate their preciousness and take steps to create an environment and conditions that encourage them to contribute fully and build a future with your organization.

Your actions reveal the value you place on your employees as well. Starting with how you orient new employees, you roll out the red carpet to communicate immediately how important they are to your team. You care deeply about hearing and responding to their concerns. When a staff member identifies a barrier that prevents doing a good job, you mobilize, running interference to remove the barrier. You understand that *you* play a powerful role in attracting and retaining talented people. Also, you realize that, in today's environment, many staff want work-life balance. Consequently you try to accommodate some of their personal needs and be considerate of their many responsibilities within and beyond work. You realize how important it is to your staff that you take pains to reduce their stress and make available the tools they require to do their jobs. You probably also realize that your staff are more likely to stay if they feel engaged, respected, appreciated, and supported.

It's a New Day

Staffing shortages abound. There are more health care jobs than qualified workers. Other providers are competing like mad for your people. Young people are not entering health care professions in sufficient numbers. The annual turnover percentage in most health care organizations has increased to double digits. The employee market is hot, and talented people call the shots (see Exhibit 10.1). The effect on people who are working in health care is enormous. They are working longer hours (mandatory overtime in some cases), with sicker, needier patients. Support systems are stretched to the bone, resources are tight, and people are doing everything they can to respond to the immediate crisis as they invest in permanent solutions.

The problem isn't limited to hospitals. Doctors' offices, ambulatory clinics, long-term care facilities, and home health agencies are experiencing similar pressure. Demographics are increasing the number of people who need health care, as baby boomers age and older people live longer. All the while, the word on the street is, "Look elsewhere for a career."

Exhibit 10.1. The Killer Question.

"Since I can work anywhere, why in the world should I work for you?"

Most health care leaders understand that the only sensible recruitment and retention strategy is to create happy employees and earn a reputation as a great place to work. There is no patient care without talented qualified staff—and enough to go around. Your success in contributing to your organization's mission depends on your having wonderful people. Your behavior as manager is powerful in retaining employees, and because your current employees spread the word, it is pivotal in recruiting employees as well.

This starts with valuing employees and not taking them for granted. There is a great difference between a leader who operates from the mind-set that employees are replaceable and dispensable and one who considers staff members as important people and precious assets. The classic statements "They should be lucky to have a job," "If they don't like it, they can go elsewhere," "My way or the highway" reveal an attitude that employees are easily replaceable, an attitude that leads to behavior and actions that push employees right out the door. No staff, no services, no organization, no future. It's that simple.

To attract really good people, you have to distinguish yourself as *a manager of choice*—someone employees respect, and someone who in turn respects and appreciates them for themselves and their contributions.

Take a Look

The difference between an employee-as-expendable attitude and one of employee-as-precious translates into how you handle everyday situations.

Raoul and Curtis

One of Raoul's employees, Curtis, approaches him, claiming unfair pay. Raoul finds such complaints frustrating, since they never cease. Acting from an employee-as-expendable attitude, Raoul promises Curtis that he will look into it but then takes weeks to get around to it. Curtis has to remind Raoul to follow up: "What's the scoop? It's been six weeks."

In contrast, thinking differently about the value of employees, Raoul responds to Curtis's concern that he isn't being paid enough by listening and asking questions. Raoul says, "Here's what I'll do to look into this with HR. . . . I'll do it this week and keep you posted on the results. You can be sure I'll follow through quickly, and I will certainly get an answer for you within two weeks. Does that sound reasonable?"

Trinh

Trinh has become aware of backbiting and finger pointing on her team. New people are swallowed up. Old-timers keep saying, "This isn't the way we do things here." It seems that staff don't give each other an inch. Angry about this and viewing employees as replaceable, Trinh takes steps to find out who the instigators are, so she can deal with them individually. She begins planning to remove them from the organization.

In contrast, seeing her employees as precious, Trinh acts differently. She decides to do all she can to salvage and resolve the situation by building her team in a variety of ways. She develops a plan to work with her diverse staff to build a mutually respectful, high-performing team in which people value one another. Until she is ready to try doing this, she decides to hold off on any efforts to focus blame on particular individuals.

Phyllis and Aletha

Phyllis is a good staff member who happens to be a single parent. One day, she asks her manager, Aletha, if she can alter her work hours to manage her kids' changing school and after-school program schedules. Thinking *There's more where she came from* and not wanting to accommodate Phyllis's individual issues, Aletha says, "Sorry, that would be inconvenient for us; it would also set a precedent. You'll need to figure out how to manage your hours and your kids without my making an exception with your schedule."

If Aletha recognizes the preciousness of her employees and the difficulty of replacing them with qualified people, she considers the fact that staff members have lives outside of work. Most are juggling work, family, and other responsibilities. Not wanting Phyllis to explore whether the hospital down the street will give her a better schedule, Aletha considers with Phyllis how to make a revised schedule work out for Phyllis and the team. She then convenes a meeting with staff members who would be affected to discuss the rationale and find out how they can all help make it work.

Alice and Richard

Alice's employee Richard is terrific at what he does. Richard approaches Alice, saying that he's tired of doing the same thing all the time and wants new challenges. Alice values Richard for what he does and regrets this request. She says in a nice way, "I'm sorry to hear that, but the job is the job. This is what we need you to do!" She is running the risk that he will find a job with new challenges elsewhere.

If she views employees as precious, she handles his request differently—and seriously. She realizes that he might leave and knows that the organization would lose out if he left. Hearing the importance to Richard of learning and growth, she asks for time to think about it and see if she can develop some diversification or stretch options for him, such as project work, committee leadership, teaming with a mentor in another part of the organization, coaching to write an article, and the like.

Alice develops alternatives and presents them to him, reiterating that her first choice is to have Richard stay in his current job with some added flexibility to do these stretch projects. If he says this is not sufficient, that he wants a different job, she offers to talk with colleagues and HR in hopes of identifying another opportunity within the organization. She tells him, "We really value you and your talent and would like to find a way for you to continue working here."

Dawn

People on Dawn's long-term care unit find themselves complaining often of a linen shortage that prevents them from providing their patients with fresh linen when they need it. Accustomed to a certain level of problems and frustration, Dawn expresses regret and annoyance, saying "it's always been that way here."

If cognizant of the preciousness of her staff and the fact that other nursing homes probably provide their caregivers with an adequate supply of linen, Dawn treats this recurrent complaint differently. She says to her team, "Even though this has been a long-standing problem, I am going to put some new energy into it, so you can get the linen you need for our patients." Dawn pursues this issue relentlessly, going to the manager of linen first, then their administrator, and then others affected by the problem. She advocates for her employees, insisting that the organization must make available the tools they need to do their jobs well.

What Worries You?

Are you overwhelmed by the complexity and scope of the issues causing people to leave the health care field? Certainly, there are many causes of job flight, many of which you cannot, as an individual manager, control.

Are you afraid of appearing ineffective in the face of the forces causing job flight? If you actively take responsibility for retaining your staff and they leave anyway, it may reflect negatively on you and your management style, unless you present yourself as powerless in the face of market forces affecting staffing.

Are you angry that, whether employees stay or leave, they have the power to make or break your team's effectiveness? Some managers fear that by communicating great appreciation to their employees, the latter will feel their oats, that they'll have too much power.

Are you afraid you don't have the creativity you need to retain your talented staff? Solutions take creative thinking on the part of all of us. You have to stick your neck out to advocate for staff needs, think outside the box, and try things that you may not have tried before.

Are you afraid of the fallout you'll face if you cater to the needs of individuals on your team? You might have to bend rules and make exceptions for the job to be workable for an individual. If you do that, you then have to handle the fallout with other staff who perceive this as unfair or a double standard. It is much simpler to have black-and-white rules.

These worries are plaguing, but managers who value employees have achieved trust and loyalty among their staff. They have helped people bond with each other and the organization and feel good about their teams. The managers themselves have benefited in the process.

What Do You Stand to Gain?

If you treat your staff members as valuable, respected people, then you, your team, your customers, and your organization all reap significant benefits.

- *By treating your staff as your organization's most precious assets, you leave your staff members feeling greater satisfaction.* They enjoy your appreciation. On a practical note, they raise fewer issues and tensions for you to address. This frees you up to attend to the strategic issues that otherwise take a back seat.

- *Staff appreciate your respect for them.* As a result, they are more likely to partner with you to meet the group's goals. They want the group to be successful, and they take ownership and pride in its success.

- *An atmosphere of mutual regard between you and the staff ripples outward to the patients.* You've no doubt been in a situation where you became tense because you could sense tension in a group. When your team coalesces and works well together, when the members help and support each other, your patients and other customers feel it. It makes them feel confidence in your team and that they are in good hands.

- *You don't have to engage in a tug of war with resistant employees.* If employees don't feel valued, they often vie for attention in negative ways—resisting your requests, moving slowly, mouthing off, and the like. If you communicate their importance, they devote more of their energy working with you, not against you. This makes your workday more harmonious.

- *Your turnover drops.* This is a big payoff. Value your employees, and they are likely to stay. Because they stay, you are likely to have adequate staffing. You have less recruitment to do, which is a relief these days when health care workers are in short supply. Because you have fewer new people to locate, interview, hire, orient, and train, you have less down time, greater productivity, and improved continuity of services. You benefit from the knowledge, skill, and teamwork of your seasoned people. What's more, calling in sick and abusing sick time diminish. Staff are more willing to cover for and help each other out if you build a supportive workteam in which everyone feels valued by you. Your longer-term employees speak positively about your team and you, instead of spreading cynicism.

- *Your staff members don't feel a need to unionize.* If you treat your staff as indispensable, listening to them and attending to their needs, they feel respected, and they have no reason to seek third-party representation.

There is so much riding on talented staff that it behooves you to elevate their importance. You reap significant benefit by treating your employees so well that they choose to cast their lot with you and your organization.

What Can You Do? How Can You Do It?

Many people think the answer lies in salary increases. It is certainly important to compensate people fairly. Though you can't underpay people if you want their satisfaction and loyalty, it is not *all* about money.

First of all, employees want to be in on things. They want the opportunity to contribute meaningfully. They want to feel involved and respected for their contribution. When they feel that no one cares what they think and that their ideas and suggestions are not respected, these are dissatisfiers.

Employees also want to be in the know. We regularly hear, "Nobody tells me anything." If you don't keep employees in the loop, they feel dispensable and devalued.

They want to do a good job. Especially in health care, employees are dedicated to serving their patients and other customers well. Facing daily obstacles that make this impossible, or suffering from not having the tools they need to do their jobs, they become understandably disheartened and wonder, "Is the grass greener at St. Elsewhere?"

Employees itch for the opportunity to learn and grow. Most people want to be successful, and they place high value on an organization that cares about and invests in helping them meet their learning needs.

Employees want to belong, to work in a supportive group. They want to feel connected to their coworkers. Given the challenges and stresses inherent in health care jobs, they rely on comfort and harmony with their coworkers.

Employees also want to be treated as individuals. They want someone to care about *their* needs and issues, to be flexible and help them meet their diverse responsibilities at work and outside. They want you to care about their well-being and their life beyond the workplace.

These are just a few of the many factors to consider. In other chapters, we share strategies that help you address several of these factors. We offer strategies you can use to build relationships with your staff, facilitate dialogue, gain an organizational perspective, help staff embrace change, and become an effective coach. All of these contribute to your becoming more effective in satisfying, gratifying, and retaining your staff.

Because we feel so strongly about this role shift, we focus here on additional strategies that help you demonstrate high regard for your employees. These strategies (Exhibit 10.2) are relatively easy to implement, and they are well within your span of control.

Exhibit 10.2. Your Employee-As-Precious Toolkit.

Strategy one: Think thoughts that support high regard for your employees.

Strategy two: Start people off on the right foot.

Strategy three: Keep tabs on employee feelings.

Strategy four: Foster bonding and belonging; create a connected team.

Strategy five: Sculpt the job; cater to the individual.

Strategy six: Remove obstacles; advocate.

Strategy seven: Communicate your regard with appreciation and thanks.

The first strategy helps you examine your belief system. It may be that you need to alter your thoughts and assumptions about your staff to treat them as the precious beings that they are.

The second strategy helps you reevaluate your new employee orientation process, revamping it as needed so that the process immediately demonstrates to new staff members how eager you are to invest in them, respect them, and create conditions that help them thrive.

The third strategy helps you keep tabs on your employees' feelings. If you are in close touch, you instinctively do a lot of the right things, because you are, after all, a caring person.

The fourth strategy is about bonding and belonging. Most people want to belong to a group. They want to feel harmony, trust, and mutual respect. If they feel these things, they are much less likely to jump ship. They feel ties that bind. By using tools to help staff members connect with one another, you can enhance these positive conditions.

The fifth strategy is about *job sculpting*, or using what you know about each employee to customize the job to the individual, building on his particular strengths, making her work schedule doable, and taking other steps to cater to them because they are precious to you.

The sixth strategy is about your role as troubleshooter and advocate for your employees. They rely on you to issue the tools and offer the support they need to do a good job. You are their lifeline. By sticking your neck out to solve problems beyond *their* control, you demonstrate the value you place on their success and well-being.

The seventh and final strategy addresses your role as communicator of esteem for your employees. By reaching new heights of generosity with thanks and appreciation, you can help your team feel the regard emanating from you.

As you can see, it is an enormous and multidimensional challenge to treat your employees as precious people who are at the same time your organization's most precious assets.

Strategy One: Think Thoughts That Support High Regard for Your Employees

We are struck with the difference in beliefs held by managers who truly value employees and their counterparts who consider employees to be interchangeable commodities. Using this first tool, examine your own thoughts and consider adjustments that align with high regard for staff.

⚒ Tool: Internal Debate

Purpose. This tool allows you to examine your own thinking; it creates arguments that increase your esteem for your employees.

Method. In the left-hand column of the grid below, you'll find beliefs commonly held by managers whose employees do not feel highly valued. These beliefs lead to management behavior and decisions that result in unnecessary turnover.

Internal Debate

Common Thought	Counterargument	Replacement Thought	Explain Why This Works
There's more where they came from!		I can't take my employees for granted.	
Employees these days don't care.		It's on me to create conditions that earn commitment.	
People's personal issues are not my concern.		My employees are people first, employees second.	
Employees are never satisfied; their complaints are management-bashing.		I'm lucky when they speak up; it gives me the chance to make course corrections.	
Job satisfaction is all about money.		I play an enormous role in my employees' job satisfaction.	
About the talent shortage, "This too shall pass."		This retention problem is not going away.	

Think about one belief at a time. Ask yourself, *Do I think this?* Whether the answer is yes or no, jot down an argument against this belief in the second column.

Next, read the alternative belief in the third column of the grid, and chew on it. Finally, jot down in the fourth column why this belief makes sense. Why is it constructive?

Adopting the beliefs on the right side of the grid may require some humility on your part, and this can be painful. But these beliefs lead you to act in ways that show your employees respect and earn their commitment.

Once you have checked your thoughts to ensure that they encourage esteem for your employees, how can you communicate this esteem effectively in your everyday management practices? Starting with first impressions, let's look at how you welcome new employees onto your team.

Strategy Two: Start People Off on the Right Foot

Do you remember what it was like to be the new kid on the block at work? You were probably excited and nervous. You wanted people to like you; you hoped to fit in. You wanted to be a success. For most of us, the seeds of satisfaction or dissatisfaction are planted during the first few days.

Mindful of this strategic opportunity, we encourage you to do what few managers do, namely, design ways to help new staff members get a flying and enthusiastic start that sets off a positive chain reaction leading to a gratifying experience on your team and in your organization.

✪ Tool: The Hearty Welcome

Purpose. This tool alerts your team to the arrival of a new employee; using it, you can plan with the team for a hearty welcome.

Method. Engage your staff in a discussion. Ask yourselves, "How do we want our new partner to feel about the work and the team? What do we want our partner to know about the work and the team?" Then build a simple plan along with them to ease the new team member's way into the group.

Here is a smorgasbord of suggestions that other teams have used successfully (Exhibit 10.3).

Exhibit 10.3. The Hearty Welcome: An Idea Smorgasbord.

Welcome basket. Fill a basket with goodies, including a card stating "How glad we are that you're here," along with "survival" items, such as Life Savers; Band-Aids; hot list (who to call for what); a map of the workspace showing where to find critical items; coupons for use in the coffee shop, cafeteria, or gift shop; and other creative options generated by your team.

Get-to-know-you-session. Arrange a staff meeting early on where you and your group introduce yourselves to the new partner. Ideas for this:

- People say one nice thing about one other person in the room
- People share who brings what to the group, focusing on something positive
- People share something they like about the team and their jobs
- People in the group get to ask the new person three questions about themselves (of course, the new person has a right to pass, and the new person gets to ask the group three questions as well)
- Everybody in the group shares something they value in their personal lives

Buddy or partner. Create a buddy system that links an experienced employee with the new employee. Let the team design all the things the buddy can do to be helpful, such as have lunch with the new employee and different members of the team daily for a week, spend time in the beginning of the day and at the end of the day talking ("What do you want to learn today? What did you learn today?"), or let the new employee watch the buddy handle sticky situations or difficult customer interactions.

Post an introduction. Invite two or three staff members to interview the new person, and take a picture and post it surrounded by things they learned about the person. Make sure they get the new person's approval before posting.

Personally devote time. Most important, be sure that you make yourself accessible and spend time with your new employee to let this person know that you are committed to helping him or her be successful. Take the employee to lunch and on a tour. Introduce the person to others, your boss, and team members. Ask how the person is feeling so far and how you can help.

You know the power of first impressions. In the fray of so much work and lean staffing, it's understandable that you would want your new employees to hit the ground running. But many report that this is exactly how it feels—as if they are hitting the ground, and that the ground is a quicksand of newness—new people, new roles, new spaces, new boss. By planning a wonderful welcoming experience, you show your regard for your employees immediately and get their relationships and performance off on the right foot.

The second strategy we suggest is tuning in to all of your employees' (not just your new employees') thoughts and feelings, so you can be responsive and caring in decisions that affect them, and in your interaction with them.

Strategy Three: Keep Tabs on Employee Feelings

Some organizations conduct employee satisfaction surveys. But a survey does not take the place of *you* taking the pulse of your team in an up-close and personal way. Here's a short report card you can use to take the pulse of your employees, regarding some of the critical success factors that affect employee commitment and retention.

⚒ Tool: Employee Pulse

Purpose. This tool is useful for finding out how your employees feel about factors over which you have some control.

Method. Circulate the report card shown in Exhibit 10.4 at least once per quarter to find out how your employees are feeling and perceiving your management effectiveness. Share the results openly with them in a meeting.

Thank people for their feedback. Show responsiveness to their perception by telling them what course corrections you want to make. Better yet, invite their suggestions. Tell them you'll be asking them to fill this out again in three months so you can see how they're doing and how you're doing.

By using a short homegrown survey of this sort, you gain valuable information about how your group feels and can then take steps to enhance their work experience and relationship with you. It is also a *safe* way to surface thoughts and

Exhibit 10.4. Employee Pulse.

My Manager . . .	Grade (A, B, C, D, or F)	My Suggestions
Has made an effort to get to know me and show respect for who I am.		
Communicates thoroughly and often, so I feel in the loop.		
Shows respect for my life outside of work.		
Shows flexibility to help me manage the many facets of my life.		
Encourages me to express my concerns and shows responsiveness.		
Helps coworkers get along, so we have harmony within our team.		
Helps me feel appreciated.		
Advocates for what we need; removes barriers.		
Finds ways to help us lighten up and have fun.		
Provides learning opportunities; helps me grow.		

feelings among your team. But some managers say, "This is too formal! Can't we just talk?" There is certainly a time for dialogue. In fact, we think it's critical that managers spend time talking to their people one-on-one. But be careful about just talking in a group setting. If only a vocal minority share their views, you run the risk of drawing lopsided conclusions.

The next tool is a great guide to one-on-one pulse taking with individuals on your team.

✪ Tool: How I Feel About My Job

Purpose. This tool helps you understand your employees and how they feel about their work, so you can use this understanding to support their success and job satisfaction.

Method. Spend time with each of your employees at least twice a year. Use the opportunity to get to know and understand your people better and gain insight into how they feel about their job. Make sure they know that you are interested in their suggestions and value their opinions. Be honest and open during the interaction, and you will get a true picture.

Here are great questions to ask:

- When do you feel you are really making a difference?
- What is the best part of your job?
- Without holding back or being embarrassed, tell me what you value most about yourself, your work, and our team.
- If you could change one thing about your job, what would it be?
- What does it feel like to be part of this team?
- If you were king or queen, what would you do to improve our team?

These conversations help you know your people. You can then act on what you know, doing all you can to make your organization a wonderful place for staff as well as for patients and other customers.

Once you have integrated new people into your group, the challenge is to build a strong, cohesive team, a connected team in which the ties between team members encourage people to stay with your organization and not be lured away for a few more dollars. The next strategy helps you build these ties that bind.

Strategy Four: Foster Bonding and Belonging; Create a Connected Team

When we ask employees what's important to them about their job, one prevalent theme that inevitably emerges is this: feeling good about their coworkers. It is no easy feat to engender coworker harmony, as teams become more diverse in terms of age, gender, nationality, race, culture, religion, sexual preference, work style, disability, learning style, and every other difference imaginable. In this atmosphere of growing diversity, connection and mutual respect within your team become all the more important to your work climate as well as to each individual's job satisfaction, loyalty, and commitment.

See how many yeses you and your group score on the short checklist in Exhibit 10.5.

Exhibit 10.5. Are We Connected?

	Yes	No
Coworkers in this group know personal things about each other.	____	____
Coworkers respect each other's ideas.	____	____
Coworkers willingly work with and support each other.	____	____
Coworkers feel responsible for each other's success.	____	____
Coworkers give each other feedback openly.	____	____
Coworkers ask each other for what they want and need.	____	____
Coworkers like to get together socially.	____	____
Coworkers laugh and have fun together at work.	____	____

If you answered no to some of these questions, don't despair. It's hard to deliberately foster great coworker relationships among your other responsibilities. The irony is that when you make the time for it, you end up saving time by increasing cooperation and support and relieving tension that otherwise drains precious energy from you and your team.

There are loads of tools available to help your people get to know each other better and to build people's esteem for themselves and others. Here's one of our favorite quick and easy bonding activities, with a big payoff.

✖ Tool: Gifts I Bring

Purpose. This tool helps build self-esteem in and among your team by recognizing the individual gifts of team members.

Method. Surprise your team in staff meetings by engaging them in this activity. Distribute the following handout to each person. Give them five minutes to check the items in which each person takes pride.

Gifts I Bring

___ 1. My ability to juggle different parts of my life

___ 2. My wonderful family

___ 3. I give honest and direct feedback.

___ 4. My many good friends

___ 5. A time I stuck my neck out courageously

___ 6. A sports accomplishment

___ 7. How I responded to a friend in need

___ 8. My nationality and family customs

___ 9. A special childhood

___ 10. My ability to express my opinions, even when at odds with others

___ 11. My good taste

___ 12. My self-discipline regarding my health

___ 13. My coworker relationships

___ 14. The values and beliefs I live by

___ 15. How I took on a challenge and handled it successfully

___ 16. My ability to balance work and play

___ 17. My energy level

This exercise exemplifies the many that are available as fun, quick ways to form team connection. Even if your staff members have been together for some time, chances are there is much more they can discover about each other. Who else but you can make this happen?

To go beyond this basic knowledge of each other and apply this to building strong work relationships, it helps to engage your staff in agreeing on a set of shared commitments about their group behavior, all with the purpose of preserving group harmony and support.

 Tool: Coworker Commitments for Workgroup Harmony

Purpose. This tool is useful for creating shared commitments that foster harmony among coworkers on your team.

Method. Ask your team to form small groups and think about teams they have been on in the past, successful and unsuccessful.

- Ask each group to make two lists: first, of behavior that supports teamwork; second, of unhelpful, destructive group behavior. After a few minutes, ask the teams to share their lists. Listen for themes that emerge.

- Ask a small group to become the wordsmiths who take the input from the small groups and prepare a draft of team commitments for the next meeting. The following list gives an example of the results from one group, the "Tower 9 coworkers."

"Tower 9 Coworkers": Commitments

1. Ask for what you want and need.
2. Respect other people's ideas and opinions.
3. Give honest and direct feedback.
4. Address problems directly, not by going behind someone's back.
5. Show up on time, so others don't have to do your work.
6. Give negative feedback respectfully.
7. Take care of our environment.
8. Listen when other people are talking.
9. Don't be a hog. Let everyone have a chance to talk.
10. Keep your promises.

Once you have commitments in place, coach your team to act with integrity toward each other in sticky situations. Managers we respect spend time helping their team learn healthy ways to keep each other on track. This next tool suggests several situations for group practice.

✪ Tool: Sticky Coworker Situations

Purpose. This tool helps you coach staff to handle sticky situations with their coworkers effectively, so strain doesn't develop and fester.

Method. Engage your group in identifying (without getting personal) sticky interpersonal situations that arise with coworkers.

Next, engage the group in generating constructive ways to handle these situations. Here are examples:

- What can you say to a coworker who arrives every day and then spends time talking about personal problems?

- You are a new employee and try to share ideas and suggestions for improvement. But a group of staff members say, "That'll never work," or "We can't ever do that here."

- One of your coworkers has spent a great deal of her personal time helping you with a difficult problem. You know this staff member went out of her way to help you, and you want her to know how much you appreciate her actions.

Divide your team into small groups, and give them five minutes to think of good ways to handle these situations. Ask, "Specifically, what would you *say*?" Compare notes in the large group. End by encouraging people to give each other constructive feedback using approaches like those shared, for the sake of the team.

These tools help you create an atmosphere where your people feel supported and safe. If people are not direct with one another, if they talk behind one another's back, they will feel alienated from coworkers, and team spirit will erode.

Don't forget the power of fun and laughter as a bonding experience that sparks team spirit. Just as ritual makes for family loyalty, so too do we need ritual at work that is "a thing apart," that respects your team by lightening their hearts. Bring in a box with all kinds of hats. In a staff meeting, invite people to grab and wear a hat that reflects their mood. We promise it will be funny, especially if you include a firefighter hat, a baseball cap, a Viking hat with horns, a few old nurse's caps, a police cap, some funny wigs, and the like.

In a staff lounge, start a cartoon bulletin board. Invite people to bring in baby pictures for a guessing game. Bring in funny toys that can relieve stress, such as rubber darts, stress balls, play dough, talking key chains, fortune-telling balls, and the like. Bring in a few dozen clown noses, or wear Groucho glasses with a mustache. Hand out ridiculous lollipops. Bring in a massage therapist with a portable chair, to give your team members ten-minute massages.

Set an atmosphere where you encourage people to laugh and do things that build good feeling and reduce stress. They will read this accurately, as respect and care for them emanating from you, and they will be right.

Strategy Five: Sculpt the Job; Cater to the Individual

Communicating regard for your employees, regard that they feel, depends increasingly on treating them as distinct individuals with their own needs, backgrounds, talents, aspirations, and expectations. The age of generic solutions to people management is gone. You have employees who differ from one another in many ways, as we have just suggested.

Take a look, for instance, at our summary in Exhibit 10.6 of generational differences that affect work attitude and decisions (gleaned from *Workforce for the New Millennium*, 2000; and "The New Workforce . . .," 2001).

Worker differences now make the strategy of customization through job sculpting an utter business necessity. It involves tailoring, customizing, designing, catering the job or conditions surrounding the job to suit the individual. This trend extends beyond your organization's pay and benefits. It extends to you and the decisions you make in your relationship and negotiation with each individual on your staff.

Before discussing the issues on which individualization has become so important, let's see how well you know your staff as individuals. Try playing a round of Work-Life-Balance Bingo (Exhibit 10.7). See if you know of an employee to whom each bingo square applies.

All of this and other work-life information affects your employees' worklife every day. Your ability to customize arrangements, solutions, motivational strategies, and work to each person depends first of all on your knowing a whole lot about each person.

Exhibit 10.6. Generational Differences.

Matures (Born 1909–1945)	Boomers (1946–1964)	Xers (1965–1983)	Generation Y: Nexters, Millennials (1977–1997)
Success over adversity; hard work; self-sacrifice	Outspoken, challenge authority; the "me" generation	Don't take anything for granted; cynical, independent	A mix: optimistic, skeptical, egocentric
Self-discipline; sense of purpose; live to work	Seeking simplicity in their work lives	Work to live; job a means to an end, not the end itself; want a job *and* a life	Community-focused; vive la différence; global consciousness
Want flexibility and stability	Seeking flexibility	Want flexibility; keep options open; live life to the fullest	Smart, show me the money, techno-savvy
Focused on family	Fixated on self-improvement	Comfort with job and career changes; modular; move easily from place to place	Want choices and custom solutions; strong family connections
Job retraining; job sharing	Seek meaning and fulfillment through work; seek achievements	Comfort with diversity	Team players, and want to be most valuable players
Self-confident; eager to share their wisdom	Want the straight scoop, the real story	Value learning and more learning; quit when they don't	Confident in future; trust in authority; pressure to excel
Want traditional training opportunities and recognition as wise elders	Want money, career advancement, and instant gratification; spend more, save less	Wary, "why me" generation, pragmatic, skeptical about institutions	Want challenge, big bucks, global opportunities

Exhibit 10.7. Work-Life-Balance Bingo.

Is involved in a legal issue	Just reached a milestone birthday	Has big debts	Wants to retire shortly	Has a big religious event coming up
Has a chronic illness	Is paying college tuition	Gets exercise every day	Recently split up with partner	Has a family member who is very sick
Is building a home or renovating	Is working full-time and going to school	Has credit card debt	Is trying to have a baby	Is planning an amazing vacation
Has trouble managing finances	Has a really plaguing teenager	Has a family member with an addiction	Has day care problems	Is strapped from paying for a wedding
Child needs after-school care	Supports an unemployed adult	Is panicky about finances	Is going through a divorce	Won an award recently

Once you know your people, stay in touch and in tune to keep learning about them. It helps to touch base with individuals, observe them at work, and talk with them, but your best hope is to ask them questions and treat what they tell you as precious gems that enable you to make their job work for them.

Strategy Six: Remove Obstacles; Advocate

Making the job work for people also requires you to become their advocate. One surefire way you can show respect for your staff is to make sure they are able to do their jobs well. Most people want to do a good job; they get frustrated if they have to jump through hoops, beg for resources, and navigate roadblocks. Out of respect and support for your staff, run interference and serve as their indefatigable advocate for what they need to do their job.

Starting with the easy problems that interfere with staff performance, here's a way to engage your team in eliminating barriers within their control.

✪ Tool: What's in the Way? (Leebov, Scott, and Olson, 1998)

Purpose. This tool identifies barriers that staff see as preventing them from performing their jobs well; the tool helps in sharing responsibility for eliminating the barriers.

Method. Begin by discussing barriers and obstacles in the broad sense. Let staff know that you are intent on eliminating obstacles to their effectiveness. Build their confidence by reminding people of barriers the group has overcome in the past.

Now, ask the group to brainstorm specific, everyday things that pose obstacles to their providing quality service to patients or other customers. As people brainstorm, write the responses on sticky notes, one barrier on each note.

Mount the stickies on the wall, and ask the group to cluster them in categories of related items (policy issues, equipment issues, people issues, team relationship issues, communication issues, systems issues, and so on). Once your team has clustered the ideas, give each small group one cluster to consider, sorting the issues into these piles:

- Quick fix: an action we can accomplish right away
- Breakthrough barrier: an accomplishment that would make a big difference if we could only figure out how to achieve it
- Unpreventable barrier: whatever we might not be able to fix, but we can develop ways to work around it or minimize its effects

Have groups present their findings. Acknowledging their precious time, ask the team to look over the quick fixes to select those they can act on immediately and those they can handle down the line:

- Why do we feel this obstacle needs to be removed?
- What will it take for us to do so?
- What support, resources, or information will we need to help us?
- What can our team expect from us, and by when?

The small groups then share their plans with the larger group, and you help them organize themselves to follow through.

Processes like this keep the attention on making improvements that ease the frustration inherent in your staff's jobs. Of course, if you are going to spend time and energy working on improvement, make sure you reap the desired effects on staff morale by helping your team savor every accomplishment. Too many people want others to believe that nothing happens here.

Keep a staff log where people can chart progress related to improvement projects. Put up a We're on the Move graffiti board and encourage people to share progress. End all meetings with a quick appreciation exercise. You'll find a great collection in our book *Achieving Impressive Customer Service* (Leebov, Scott, and Olson, 1998).

Your team can achieve some quick fixes without involving others in the organization, but many barriers to their doing a good job lie beyond walls of your domain. What about when nurses don't have enough linen delivered on time? Or when no patient education materials are available to support the nurse's predischarge discussion with the patient and family? What about when the food warming system is inadequate, and food servers hear daily complaints about hot food arriving cold? What about when a secretary cannot get approval to buy a computer with enough memory to handle the jobs you ask that secretary to do?

These are just a few examples of obstacles to doing a job that make employees crazy and cause them to question their importance. What's the solution? If you consider your employees to be indispensable, then as they endure obstacles that go beyond their control you must act as a tireless advocate for what they need to be successful.

You can overcome some of their obstacles by setting your mind to it with determination the likes of which they have never before seen. You can make something important happen by taking on the issue with a vengeance.

In some cases, you will be wise to form teams or pressure individuals to hold up their end—to provide the services and supports on which your folks rely to do their job. This often means you have to initiate courageous conversation with your boss or colleagues in other departments. Shifting from silo thinking to an organizational perspective, you must cross lines and raise issues boldly, insisting that solutions are a must for the sake of the organization's mission. In Chapter Six, on building relationships, one of the tools we shared is the partnership contract, which can help you address those obstacles beyond your walls that are oppressive to your staff.

Some fixes really are out of your control. Exhibit 10.8 has tips on how to be an effective advocate as your people are awaiting a change or an answer.

Exhibit 10.8. Advocacy Tips.

- *Give the straight scoop.* Let your staff know honestly what you can and can't do, and why. Don't ever say "I'll ask" or "I'll take care of that" unless you mean it.

- *Respond with urgency.* When your people raise concerns, they feel them urgently. Mirror the urgency they feel, and follow up without delay.

- *Follow up tenaciously.* Tell your staff what you intend to do, how you will get back to them, and by when. People hate feeling as if their ideas and requests have entered a deep pit. Even if you don't have the answers, let people in on the process.

- *Hold an open forum.* Bring your boss in to your area to talk with and listen to your people. Help your staff form questions beforehand, encouraging them to raise real issues. Coach people to ask these questions constructively, so they are less likely to receive a defensive response.

- *Arrange leadership rounds.* Make sure your boss gets to see firsthand the issues or conditions frustrating your team.

- *Arrange job shadowing.* Try doing people's jobs yourself. You gain great respect for what your people have to do and enhance fervor and credibility when you approach your boss or colleagues to initiate improvement.

These tips help you keep the faith with your employees while you advocate for them and address their unspoken question, "Could someone here possibly care about us?"

Going to bat for your people often happens behind the scenes. They realize you did it when you present a solution. The last strategy we want to suggest is an up-close and personal one, namely, seeing to it that you generously give each person *individualized* appreciation and thanks.

Strategy Seven: Communicate Your Regard with Appreciation and Thanks

You've undoubtedly been lectured about this more times than you can count. Here we go again. Wendy ran some focus groups for a big hospital system that wanted to reevaluate its many reward and recognition systems. This system had numerous methods in place and felt the need to sort through them, eliminate those that didn't work, and strengthen the overall approach. In group after group, after listing more than thirty recognition methods going on in that system, Wendy asked people to identify those with the biggest impact. One hundred percent of the people picked just one approach. The most powerful approach, said each and every person, is "a pat on the back from my supervisor." They said that this one approach, one of the few that cost not one penny, was the rarest of all.

In short, if you want your employees to feel precious to you, call them by name. Inquire about how they're doing. Notice and appreciate them. Compliment them about specific things that they do well and specific ways they contribute. Credit them for their accomplishments. Give this positive regard whether you're getting it from *your* boss or not. Acknowledge big life events. Send an occasional compliment to them at their home address, so they're sure to show it to their family.

Find one way after another to express high regard to them directly. Any high regard you think you have for them is invisible unless you express it.

Employees on a Pedestal

The shift from viewing the employee as expendable to viewing the employee as indispensable and precious may be disconcerting because it upsets the traditional feeling of authority most of us have in our management jobs. It can feel maddening that employees—in a time of shortage—seem to have us over a barrel. We have to just let go of these feelings and recognize that health care really is about valuable human beings caring for vulnerable human beings. It is the work of the soul. Shortage or not, health care employees have always deserved to be admired and supported in their caring work. It is our job to create caring communities that help them flourish.

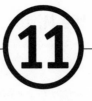

From Pressure and Overwork to Balance and Perspective

Our increasingly turbulent industry, the accelerating speed of modern life, and our multiple roles and demands have created an atmosphere of overwork and pressure. Shifting from the frenzied mode that this creates to achieve balance and perspective instead is an enormous challenge. Whether you focus on your own health and peace of mind or on how you can add the greatest value to your organization, it is a compelling necessity.

A Revealing Look in the Mirror

True or False?	True	False
1. I understand that in today's environment my work is rarely "finished." I am learning to live with this.	_____	_____
2. I have learned healthy ways to relieve pressure and stress.	_____	_____
3. I work hard to create balance in my life.	_____	_____
4. I work hard to stay focused on key priorities and not get off course with daily interruptions.	_____	_____
5. I limit the work I take home evenings and weekends.	_____	_____
6. The pressures at work are threatening my health.	_____	_____
7. My staff may very well describe me as frenzied.	_____	_____
8. I do loads of work that I wish my direct reports would do, but I can't really trust them to do these things right or by the deadline involved.	_____	_____
9. I say yes to everything my boss asks of me.	_____	_____
10. I get so preoccupied with work that I have trouble concentrating on my family and friends.	_____	_____

If you answered false to most of these statements, you are managing your time in a way that allows you a satisfying degree of balance and perspective. Most likely, you have some peace of mind and freedom from anxiety. It might mean that you do not have lots to do, but in this day and age that's unlikely. Even if you're juggling a lot of balls, you must be juggling in a way that leads to balance and perspective.

If you answered true to most of the statements, you are probably feeling overworked and oppressed by the pressures of your work. You may go home from work relieved but not gratified, tired but not feeling accomplished. You probably find yourself trying to figure out how to get a grip on all you feel you have to do. We daresay, you may also be wondering how in the world you can have more time and energy for your relationships, relaxation, and other beyond-work activities that you yearn to enjoy.

If you feel overworked and pressured, join the crowd. These frustrations are the beef of countless lunch conversations every day—if people can even make time for lunch, that is. They would be a gold mine for therapists, if those of us in this state could even find the time to squeeze a therapist into our already chock-full schedules.

It's a New Day

Pressure and overwork have crept up on us in health care leadership jobs. The health care environment has intensified and become increasingly turbulent and challenging. Our competitors are more aggressive. Consumers are more demanding. Resources are frustratingly limited. Qualified employees are disillusioned with health care and leaving in droves to pursue other careers. We've risen to the occasion by stepping up our activity, embracing multiple priorities at once, taking on increasing responsibility, and trying to do it all rapidly and well to help our organization survive and thrive.

Health care managers nationwide feel they're working like dogs and enduring the stress of multiple (if not wholly unreasonable) demands. Organizations where this is not the case are considered asleep at the wheel. Pressure and overwork have crept up on us, and many of us now feel oppressed by it beyond toleration.

But here's the rub. Just because it's the norm to feel overwhelmed and to work very, very hard and for long hours, it doesn't mean this is healthy. It doesn't mean you *like* your life with work consuming so much of your time, lifeblood, and spirit. Many of us accomplish a great deal, but it takes a personal toll. Others of us are distracted or debilitated by the feelings of pressure and fatigue, and our attention scatters and makes us inefficient and ineffective. In both cases, whether we accomplish a lot or not, we tend to feel drained and maybe even inadequate: "No matter what I do, it's never enough."

The good news is this: there *are* leaders who have found ways to maintain balance and perspective—leaders who have been able to prioritize and enforce their work and life priorities, with themselves and others. They focus their team on what's most important. Sometimes they say no to people—even to the boss. They have a life beyond work. They take breaks. They enjoy themselves. Even when things go wrong at work, they let it go and concentrate on their friends and family. Their self-worth does not depend exclusively on their work accomplishments or how many hours they spend working.

Given the insanity of our turbulent environment, industry, and world, the fiscal constraints, and the frenzy to outsprint the competition, finding balance and perspective is an enormous challenge, whether you focus on your own health and peace of mind or on how you can add the greatest value to your organization.

Would you like to feel more gratified by your accomplishments, more respected at work for your contributions, healthier, and better able to say in good conscience to friends, "I have a life"?

Take a Look

Consider these instructive cases.

Jody

Jody is manager of human resources. She reports to the CEO. Because of the talent shortage, she feels she's drowning in alligators, trying one strategy after another and doing this without having any staff other than those doing the everyday transactions of HR. Highly motivated and results-oriented, Jody implements many tactics at once, and she is swamped! On top of that, nearly every day, her boss is in and out of her office asking her to do other things.

It's Wednesday, and her boss walks in with yet another request. In a mode of overwork and pressure, Jody's habit is to think, *Darn, I really wanted to work on our retention plan, but he's my boss and I have to do what he wants.* She says, "Sure, no problem." Her boss leaves satisfied, while she stews. She thinks *Well, there goes what's important to me!*

Superwoman that she is, she produces the information for her boss, even though she is falling further behind on the retention plan and feeling very anxious about that.

If Jody were operating from a position of balance and perspective, she would act differently—with a contrasting result. Picture this: she hears her boss out and then says, "To do that for you, I will need to set aside what I'm now doing, which is really important to the organization." She then explains and negotiates. Calmly, she moves the conversation to a discussion of tradeoffs that will relieve the pressure to do it all.

Harry

On Sunday night, Harry pulls out a bunch of sticky notes from his briefcase and uses them to make a long to-do list for the week. He then looks at his calendar and sees that his week is packed with one meeting after another. Operating in a pressure-and-overwork mode, he says to his daughter, "This week's going to be hectic. I'm swamped with meetings even before I get hit with the crises. I don't think I'll be able to get to your baseball game later." His blood pressure surges and he feels an intense pang of guilt, as his daughter glares at him.

Harry lets others determine how he spends his time, and he pays a personal price for it. By the end of the week, he feels increasingly pressured, overworked, and frustrated, because he will not have accomplished what's most important to him.

In a mode of balance and perspective, Harry responds differently. Previewing his week on Sunday, he sees blocks of time allocated to his most important priorities, including time for meetings, project work, and reflection. He has already scheduled his time to ensure progress, even if in small steps, related to his priorities. What happened to all of those meetings? He got selective, or he found others to represent him, or he handled some of the business through e-mail or phone calls. Harry thinks to himself, *I can do this. My week is manageable!* He relaxes to enjoy the eleven o'clock news. Then, when Monday comes, he sticks to his schedule with minor alterations and makes it to his daughter's game.

Paul

Paul manages a service department. Over the last few months, he has been feeling particularly exhausted and has endured repeated headaches. In the habit of keeping a stiff upper lip, he suffers through them and keeps up his incessant work pace. His wife expresses concern about his health. Paul is secretly concerned, too, but he gets absorbed in his work pressure and buries those fleeting thoughts about what might be happening to him.

Desperate to break him out of this work, work, and more work mode, his wife suggests that they throw caution to the wind and go away for a long, quiet weekend. Operating from a well-established lifestyle of pressure and overwork, Paul makes excuses, insisting that if he goes away he'll be even more anxious and prone to illness.

If, however, he dedicates himself to achieving balance and perspective, he might still work like a madman occasionally. But in the face of his wife's concern, he would give a resounding yes to the idea of getting away for a long weekend.

What Worries You?

The thought of crossing the bridge from overwork and pressure to balance and perspective raises several concerns for managers in a pressure-and-overwork lifestyle.

When you think about shifting from overwork and pressure to balance and perspective, do you have concerns?

Are you a manager who likes the fray? Perhaps you feel important, indispensable, and even heroic as it is, and you're afraid you might lose that. Perhaps you believe that your long hours and high activity level win you respect and a superhero image, both of which you enjoy.

Are you afraid you'll have to say no to people? If you're one who prefers to avoid conflict, you might worry that to gain balance and perspective you would have to say no to people's requests, producing anxiety and risking the disapproval of the person making the request. You might fear that others will stop thinking of you as a team player, or see you as bringing down the team or not holding up your end.

Are you concerned that you'll be held more accountable if you appear in control of your work? If you decide on your priorities and act on them, you may feel committed to results that you're afraid you can't achieve. You won't have the excuse of overwork as the reason you can't achieve them.

Does frenzied absorption in your work help you avoid things that may be painful or unsettling in your life, such as job dissatisfaction, relationship issues at home, and more? Perhaps you are consuming yourself with your work to hide from hard issues. If you continue to work your fingers to the bone, you can avoid facing health issues that you don't want to face. Maybe, if you wear yourself out severely enough, you'll get sick and won't have to *decide* to leave a job you can't stand. The decision will be made for you.

Are you making your staff crazy? If they told you the truth, they would say you appear out of control, harried, and unapproachable, and they feel the spillover onto them. Wanting to be your salvation or gain your approval, some staff then also work harder than is healthy for them and resent it, while others work less hard because they know you'll feel responsible and fill the gaps.

Do you have a hard time relaxing even when you want to? It's hard to do. When you get home, you crash, lacking energy for loved ones and your avocations. If your family or friends resent this, you have to deal with their anger and disappointment—adding even more pressure on you. How could this *not* affect your health?

Ironically, working like a nut reaps benefits for managers who do it, which is why they express many concerns about crossing the bridge to balance and perspective.

What Do You Stand to Gain?

Look at the other side of the story. If you cross the bridge from overwork and pressure to balance and perspective, you reap precious benefits related to your health, efficiency, effectiveness, staying power, and sense of accomplishment.

- *You know what's important, and this guides you.* You feel centered and trust your own decisions.
- *You can concentrate even when your tasks are hard.* Your head doesn't spin with overload.
- *Your colleagues and boss see you as clear-headed and effective.* You accomplish important things that earn you the respect of your staff, colleagues, higher-ups, and customers.
- *You have time.* Because you are thinking about what you most want and because you are consciously choosing this, you have time to pursue learning opportunities and also time to relax and allow yourself some fun. This gives you more staying power when work presents inevitable frustration.
- *You can enjoy your life outside of work and attend to your health.* You're a role model for staff of a person with work-life balance. You stop thinking, *There must be more to life than work.* You are much more likely to engage in the things you need to do to maintain your health and peace of mind, such as exercising, eating well, playing, caring about others, and showing your loving self to your family. The result: you live longer, and your quality of life improves.

What Can You Do? How Can You Do It?

Would you be satisfied to have your tombstone read "Worked his fool head off" or "Lived for the organization and made an amazing contribution, even though her family feels they never knew her"?

There are hundreds of guides filled with zillions of methods for time management, stress management, improving spiritual and emotional health, and the like. We recommend four strategies to help you enter the blissful zone of balance and perspective (Exhibit 11.1).

The first strategy helps you examine your thinking to make sure it supports movement toward balance and perspective. Frequently, our thoughts contribute to the frenzy that we feel when under pressure.

Exhibit 11.1. Your Balance and Perspective Toolkit.

Strategy one: Address your personal attitudinal blocks.

Strategy two: Learn to identify your priorities, and do it regularly.

Strategy three: Adopt a routine of scheduling your priorities into your life.

Strategy four: Be a living example of work-life balance.

The second strategy helps you pinpoint your priorities. It helps you take into account not only what's urgently pressing but also what is most important. People who overdo the urgent and constantly postpone the important end up feeling frustrated and dissatisfied.

The third strategy helps you build your priorities into your life, since priorities without time devoted to them lead to frustration and an even greater feeling of pressure. This strategy is an approach to scheduling that ensures balance and also time dedicated to what's important to you.

The final strategy helps you consider the powerful impact you can have on your staff by becoming a role model of work-life balance. By taking on the goal of becoming a role model, you make strides in work-life balance in your life, while being inspirational for the sake of your team as well.

Strategy One: Address Your Personal Attitudinal Blocks

If you want to change from a pressure-and-overwork mode to one of balance and perspective, take a good hard look at your thoughts—your inner talk, that incessant monologue running through your head as you go about your business and your life. If you yearn for balance and perspective but don't have it now, you are probably talking to yourself and thinking thoughts that keep you where you are.

This path takes you first to a sort of swap meet, where you trade in your current thoughts for ones that are more effective in helping you achieve balance and perspective. If you can change your self-talk, this will trigger changes in your feelings and actions to achieve better work-life balance.

✖ Tool: Be Your Own Thought Architect

Purpose. This tool is useful for redesigning your thinking so that it supports balance and perspective.

Method. On a sheet of paper, make three columns. Name the left-hand column "current thoughts," the middle column "consequences," and the right-hand column "alternative thoughts."

- Under "current thoughts," list those you have about your work and yourself when you're working too hard and feeling tremendous pressure. Read them a few times, and feel the weight you're carrying when you think these thoughts. In the middle column, jot down the main consequence of each thought.

- It's time to get creative! Imagine that you're the architect of your thoughts. Renovate them so that they better support balance and perspective. Start with your first current thought and its consequences. Figure out an alternative that would help you reach your goal related to greater balance and perspective. It may help if you read the thought on the left and argue with it, to come up with your better alternative.

Exhibit 11.2 shows how a completed list might look.

- Next, dedicate yourself to the demise of your current unhelpful thoughts whenever they creep into your busy, busy brain. Become your own thought police. Tell yourself *Stop!* Then consciously select and say to yourself the alternatives you crafted to be more helpful.

- Reread your list of alternatives ten times, imprinting them on your brain.

- One last suggestion: go public. Share your goal with a close colleague or family member. Ask them to help you catch yourself when you're frenzied, reminding you of the ways of thinking that help you achieve perspective.

Even if you think your thoughts are under great control, you can reinforce your newly helpful thoughts using the powerful skill Wendy coined as "ligging" (as in *let it go*). This is a precious gem of an approach. You won't want to miss out on this one.

Exhibit 11.2. Renovating Your Thoughts.

Current Thoughts	Consequences	Alternative Thoughts
"I've got to do this—and everything—perfectly."	You exhaust yourself, and you spend more time on less important things.	"I need to pick and choose when perfection is appropriate, or I'll have no time for my enthusiasms!"
"I can't say no."	You end up spending your precious time on things other people want from you, but not what you want for yourself.	"I need to assert my priorities and negotiate."
"I've got to do this myself. I can do this best."	Maybe you can do this best, but you are overloading yourself beyond a point that's healthy.	"If I do others' jobs, I won't have time for mine."
"I'll work on my priorities later."	You may never get to the point of working on them.	"Now is the time for my priorities. 'Later' will never come."
"People won't respect me if I don't work really long hours."	You're paying a personal price working such long hours; many people think you're foolish.	"It's results, not hours, that earn respect."
"I'll focus better on the tough things if I get these little things out of the way."	The little things fill up your time, and you never get to the tough things.	"The little things will consume all of my time, if I let them."

Would people say you have a heavy sense of responsibility? We imagine you think thoughts such as *I should do this; if I don't, who will? If I don't, will others be stuck with it? How can I leave this undone when I can do it? I must take care of this; people expect it of me.* If you do, you are probably taking on work that others should be doing but are not, or tasks that are not clearly anyone's responsibility. As a result, you become overloaded and resentful. Meanwhile, the people who should be doing the work are sipping coffee, playing racquetball, going home early, watching TV, and having a life.

Ligging to the rescue! Ligging can help you prevent your heightened sense of responsibility from overtaking your life, such that you lose perspective and work yourself into the ground.

Ligging is, as we suggested, a shorthand reminder to let others do their jobs and stop yourself from filling the gaps they leave. It stands for *let it go*. Wendy's circle of friends and coworkers now know to say *lig* to Wendy when she's taking on the world and losing her balance. At the mere mention of the word, Wendy breathes deeply and lets go, thinking the helpful thoughts she knows she most needs to think.

 Tool: "Ligging"

Purpose. This tool helps you catch yourself having thoughts that lead to frustration and pressure in the face of tasks beyond your control or outside of your scope of responsibility; it allows you to stop this thinking by consciously using the shorthand "lig."

Method. List the reasons it's unhealthy for you to do other people's jobs. Is it because you won't have time for what matters most to you? Will you resent the fact that they are getting paid for what you are doing? Commit to telling yourself to *lig* (let it go) when you are about to take on someone else's responsibility because you want to help, or you don't trust the person to do it, or because the person is resisting it.

- Now, list the reasons it's unhealthy for you to be upset and pressured when the source of this is beyond your control. Commit to telling yourself to lig when you're upset, angry, or frustrated about things going on at work that you cannot influence or control.

- Tell two close colleagues about your commitment to lig in these two situations. Ask them to say *lig* to you if they see or hear evidence of taking on too much or upsetting yourself unnecessarily or futilely.

Ligging works especially well when you feel stuck with something over which you don't even have complete control. You tell yourself to let it go, and you move on with the things you can control. If you become (or are already) a good ligger, you will conserve your own energy and have an easy-to-use way to restore peace of mind in the face of stress.

Strategy Two: Learn to Identify Your Priorities, and Do It Regularly

The next strategy is all about how you manage the big *P*: priorities. You need a firm grip on your priorities to make energy and attention available for them. If you react to needs and demands without a strong sense of what's most important, you may get a lot done, but not necessarily the things that matter most. Then, since those important things remain on the back burner, they eat away at you in the form of pressure and overwork. Also, if you aren't clear about what your priorities are, no wonder the tendency to work, work, work! You're in a mode of trial and error. Having lost touch with priorities, you're just working hard. When you feel that everything is a priority, this is a sign that you are out of touch with your priorities.

This second strategy helps you to prioritize, so that you can make conscious and wise decisions about how you spend your time. Then, when you spend your time that way, you get more satisfaction from your accomplishments and feel less frustration as a result.

One key to setting your priorities is to distinguish between things that are urgent and things that are important. Frequently, activities that are urgent are not important, but since they are urgent, you do them first. Also, activities that are important are frequently not urgent, so you put these important things on the back burner because you don't feel pressure to do them.

What does this have to do with perspective? Doing urgent but unimportant things demonstrates that you have lost your perspective. By making a conscious selection about what you do, considering both urgency and importance, you regain your perspective and can balance the short-term and long-term priorities facing you.

Try this next tool to help you sort out the tasks and challenges facing you.

⚒ Tool: Your Urgency-Importance Matrix

Purpose. This tool helps you sort the tasks facing you according to their urgency and importance, so you can focus more often on what's most important.

Method. Get a pad of small sticky notes. Make a no-holds-barred list of all the things you want or need to accomplish at work, big and little, urgent and long-term, voluntary initiative and command performance. Write one on each sticky note. On a table or wall, label four spaces as shown below.

Urgent, Important, or Both?

Urgent and Important	Urgent, Not Really Important	Not Urgent and Not Important	Not Urgent but Important
Budget due; customer complaint	Doing written update for your boss	Reading mail, attending meetings to appear involved	Employee coaching; planning a long-term project

Think about each sticky-note activity and move it to the appropriate heading. Drawing on what you know about your personal patterns and reflecting rationally for a moment, consider which categories should most constructively consume your time. Set a goal for yourself, as shown below.

My Goal

My Goal: Knowing me, here's what I need to do:

1. I need to spend more of my time on activities in the _____ category.

2. To free up time to do more in that category, I need to spend less of my time in the _____ category.

Use the four-category system above weekly to consciously dedicate time to your priorities.

It's really hard, but critical, to preserve the lion's share of your time for important things, whether they are urgent or not. Now, you're probably thinking, *But I've got to do the urgent, unimportant things!* That may be true in many cases, but make sure you do those things during a time when you are not functioning at peak. Do your important things during your peak time.

This next strategy helps you go beyond knowing what your priorities are, to actually *living* them. Specifically, it helps you schedule your time around your priorities. If you don't consciously schedule your priorities into your life, you'll devote to them only whatever time you have left over after you do the easy things, or the things others expect of you.

Strategy Three: Adopt a Routine of Scheduling Your Priorities into Your Life

If you see yourself as aware of your priorities but lacking the time to work on them, you are probably frustrated and want to make some changes to preserve your health. Maybe you've heard what the optimist said to the sourpuss: "If you think you're cheerful, please tell your face!" In this case, the cool cat says to the workaholic, "You may know your priorities, but tell your schedule!" Thinking some things are a priority but allocating your time in a way that is out of sync with priority is crazy-making.

The next tool helps you achieve balance and perspective, not by default but *by design.* Specifically, it entails an approach to scheduling that ensures having time available for your priorities.

⚒ Tool: Scheduling Your Priorities

Purpose. This tool helps you reserve and protect time you can use to pursue your priorities.

Method. Whether quarterly, monthly, weekly, or daily, adopt this approach to scheduling:

- List your priorities (picking up the kids on time, writing the process improvement plan, meeting with staff to discuss customer feedback, and so on).

- Identify the steps involved in working on each one. For instance, do you need to convene a group to crystallize the process improvement approach, develop a monitoring device, draft the plan, get feedback on it, revise the plan based on feedback, or whatnot?

- Decide which steps to complete within the upcoming time period. To use an example, let's say you need to schedule an up-front meeting in the first week, so you can get the group's input.

- Schedule time to work on these steps *before* you allow your calendar to fill up with other commitments. In other words, build your priorities into your calendar before you let other, less important things devour it.

You're probably saying, "But things inevitably arise that I didn't anticipate!" Yes, you must make an occasional on-the-spot decision about whether to allow any of these emerging time-consumers to take the place of your priority activity. In many situations, you have to be flexible and change your plans. The key rule is this: if you are going to do something other than the priority activity you planned to do, you must move the priority activity to another time slot within the same time period. You must *reschedule* it, *not* eliminate it.

Focusing your time and attention on your priorities, you'll find you get more satisfaction from your activities, and this helps you keep your perspective. When you devote your time to less important things, your priorities gnaw at you and make you feel pressured.

Another way you can design balance into your life is by allocating time to each of the various roles you play in your life, and stubbornly insisting that you preserve time for each role. Are you a parent, a partner, a manager, a friend, a mentor, a son or daughter, a coach, a spiritual person? Do you pay disproportionate attention to one role in your life—say, your role as manager—while shortchanging other roles in your life, such as partner or parent? Do you work so much that you don't have time to spend with your family or friends, or on avocational interests?

Try using this next tool to create balance among the many hats you wear.

⚒ Tool: Role Scheduling for Work-Life Balance

Purpose. This tool helps dedicate quality time to each role important to you in your life.

Method. Start by thinking about the roles you play in your life that are important to you. In the left-hand column of the following chart, list the *six most important roles* you play in your life (examples: manager, carpenter, baseball coach, mother, daughter, activist).

In the right-hand column, write in one or two priority activities related to each role. For instance, related to your manager role, a priority might be to "tour the team work area and connect with each individual." Related to your carpenter role, a priority might be to "make a deck." Related to your role of mother, your priority might be to "call my daughter at a time when I'm free to talk, to check on her pregnancy." Related to your role as activist, a priority might be attending a strategy meeting with fellow activists.

My Most Important Roles

Six Most Important Roles in My Life	Priority Activity Within Each Role
1. (example) Manager	(example) Walk around work areas; connect with individual staff
2.	
3.	
4.	
5.	
6.	

Insert into your actual schedule at least one priority activity related to *each* role *each week.* If there is an optimal time for a type of activity, schedule it then. In the manager example, you might schedule yourself on Wednesday at 5:30 P.M. to walk through one specific area, during the evening shift, to connect with staff in that area.

In the carpenter example, you might schedule yourself on Tuesday morning at 7:00 A.M. to go to the home supply store to pick up the lumber and supplies you need to build the foundation for the deck. In the mother example, you might write into your calendar a phone call to your daughter at 5:15 P.M. on Thursday, when you can close your door and have some peace (along with a lower phone rate).

Here's an example of how the whole chart might look.

Fitting My Roles into My Schedule

Six Most Important Roles in My Life	Priority Activity for This Role	Schedule into My Week
1. Life partner	Have meaningful nonwork conversation	Out to dinner Friday night; at Monday dinner, discuss thirty-minute limit on dinner-table discussion of work
2. Mom	Call to check on daughter's well-being at least twice a week	Call on Wednesday and Sunday before dinner, California time
3. Manager	Develop staff recruitment and retention plan	Reserve Tuesday afternoon to draft plan; meet with Lynne Wednesday to review and fix
4. Daughter	Weekly phone and e-mail contact with Mom	E-mail Monday, Wednesday, Friday; call Sunday
5. Spiritual person	Peaceful time to myself	Tuesday, Thursday evenings; Saturday morning
6. Health enthusiast	Exercise	Monday, Wednesday, Saturday before dinner

By checking yourself to make sure you are explicitly allocating time to your important roles, you maintain balance in your life. If you take for granted that you will attend to these roles and schedule yourself only for your work, then your work will grow and grow, expanding to consume disproportionate space in your life and smothering other activities that give your life meaning.

Strategy Four: Be a Living Example of Work-Life Balance

A fourth strategy that supports balance and perspective involves deciding to become a role model of work-life balance, one who shows others the way. As a leader, you influence lots of people. They look to you to set standards. They look to you as they make career decisions. They look to you as they form their aspirations. If you are a workaholic who has no life beyond work, this is your legacy to your staff. Some will respond by thinking *Wow, that way of life is not for me* and consider taking their talent somewhere that allows them to have a life. Others will follow your lead, thinking that the pattern you are demonstrating gets rewarded here, and if they want to advance as you have then they must live and work that same way.

We are kidding ourselves if we think we successfully attract young pups to health care so they can work their fingers to the bone and have no life outside of work. If you look at lifestyle trends among generation Xers, gen Yers, and nexters, you see that they consistently strive for work-life balance. When they see the work patterns of the boomers and their elders, they shriek "Not for me!" Most do not want to commit to an organization that drains their lifeblood. They would rather make less money and have the flexibility to pursue their interests and passions.

If you are plagued by stress and overwork, consider seriously a course correction. Use this tool to help you think it through.

⚒ Tool: Self-Reflection on Work-Life Balance

Purpose. This tool is useful in considering how you can benefit from work-life balance and how you might proceed.

Method. Consider these questions:

- To what extent are you plagued by imbalance between your life and work?

- What are the consequences for you? for your family? for your staff?

- What would work-life balance entail for you? Would you more often say no to urgent work if it displaced nonwork activities important to you? Would you consider time-outs, breaks, and social conversations at work as a priority, not a luxury? Would you take a few days off to go visit your grandchildren and then proudly show pictures from your trip to your coworkers without feeling guilty about taking time off? Would you actually sit down and have lunch or take a walk at midday? Would you devote short bits of time in meetings to helping people connect personally, instead of lasering in on the task with not a minute to spare?

The overwork and pressure of today's health care environment can make you and others around you nuts. Cut yourself a break; stop for lunch. Have a social conversation with a colleague. Stare out the window. Close your door and put your head down for a few minutes. Don't hesitate to laugh every chance you get.

Dedicate yourself to a breakthrough toward work-life balance. Perhaps you'll feel even more motivated if you think about the great effect your success at work-life balance could have on your team's work-life balance and the job satisfaction and appreciation that result.

✴ Tool: Be a Work-Life-Balance Role Model

Purpose. This tool helps inspire your staff to pursue work-life balance through your personal example.

Method. Tell your staff that you're working on achieving better work-life balance—and tell them how and why.

Talk about the benefits for them of work-life balance in their lives. Acknowledge the many roles they juggle in their lives, and empathize with how difficult it must be for them to work hard, have a family, go to school, be responsible for elders, and so much more.

Communicate these messages:

- I am more than my job, and so are you.
- I can set limits on my work, so that I have a life, and so can you.
- I deserve a break during the day to relax and refresh, and so do you.
- There's more to life than work for me and for you.
- It's healthy, for all of us, to have fun at work.

Close by inviting them to feel free to raise work-life balance issues for you and the team. Assert that you want them to feel their lives are manageable, even as the organization benefits from their services.

We think it's time for heroics on work-life balance. Lots of us have lost our balance, and this sends an unhealthy message to the talented people who enter a health care profession. Now is the time, for our own health, and for the present and future health and well-being of generations we influence, to clear a new path, showing people how to honor their whole being in their life and work.

It's All About Conscious Choices

Embedded in all of these strategies are an underlying theme and an alert. You won't gain balance and perspective if you are living your life unconsciously. Even if you are conscious about the decisions you make, you won't achieve balance and perspective if you just eliminate things that you're doing so as to make your life less of a rat race. The key to balance and perspective is finding your real priorities—the *meaning* in what you're doing—and consciously dedicating energy and time to the parts of your work and life that have meaning.

To figure out priorities, you need to ask, "Of all the alternatives open to me that could consume my precious lifeblood, what is important? Where do I get meaning? Where do I add value?" There are quality-of-work and quality-of-life decisions you must inevitably face. When you do, it becomes that much easier to refashion your schedule to spend your time in a way that allows you to connect with your staff and your loved ones meaningfully, and gain gratification from it.

If you succumb to overwork and pressure, you are robbing yourself of the most important parts of your life, and this can't help but have a cumulative negative impact on your leadership, your relationships, your efficiency and effectiveness, your health, your longevity, and the meaning you find in your life and work.

Isn't it ironic that, especially in health care, managers and staff alike are engaging in unhealthy overwork in an atmosphere of unrelenting pressure? Here we are, dedicated to elevating the health status of people in our communities, while we ourselves are falling apart at the seams from the stress of our work.

The strategies discussed here hold promise for liberating you from overwork and helping you discover and maintain work-life balance. By having the guts to pursue these strategies, by becoming a trailblazer, you can show others the way. You can contribute to creating healthier work environments and healthier organizations, while enhancing your own health and life beyond work. What a great epidemic this would be!

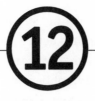

Becoming the Indispensable, Gratified Manager

These days, if you feel total mastery of your job, it's cause for suspicion. The challenges of competition, growth, financial stability, and customer satisfaction are moving targets that continuously pose new challenges to you as leader. No one has it mastered.

As we have been asserting in this book, the journey to personal mastery is lifelong. We hope we have inspired you to stretch your thinking and your repertoire of skills, so you can exemplify the ten roles so vital to becoming increasingly indispensable to your organization and ever more gratified in your job. We hope as well that you are itching to apply some of these tools right away. If so, wonderful! That is our intention.

You can go the next step by reflecting, sharing, and exploring these new skills in depth. But this exploration requires active pursuit on your part (see the example in Exhibit 12.1). Without a proactive approach to learning, your plans and books gather dust on the shelf; your vision of becoming a stronger, more skillful, more dynamic, more effective manager becomes an idle wish, a good intention. What do we mean?

Exhibit 12.1. The Buffalo Jumpers Club.

"Every now and then, I wake up out of a dream, and I'm running in front of this herd of stampeding buffaloes, and I'm running as fast as I can, and thinking to myself, 'If I could only jump high enough so I could just get out of their way. . . .'"

This dream was related by a leader in his field to a group of people he felt close to at a workshop. Later, he found that others actually had similar dreams, so they formed a "buffalo jumpers club." It was their metaphor for leadership.

"A bystander would think that I'm leading the herd of buffalo," he said. But his fellow club members all identified with the feeling that they were running just to stay ahead of the stampeding pack.

Our traditional view of leadership revolves around this image of the leader being out there, out front. Leaders usually get to where they are by knowing the answer. Our leaders are supposed to not only know more than those behind them but also know the right answer.

That puts a leader in a very difficult spot. . . . We know that we learn by doing, and in that learning we are going to make mistakes. Making mistakes makes it quite obvious that we don't know what it is we're learning about—and for leaders, that's a dilemma.

In the new model of leadership, the leaders are still supposed to be out front, but now they are supposed to be out there making mistakes faster than anyone else.

Source: Kim (1997), p. 33. Reprinted from *Healthcare Forum Journal,* vol. 36, no. 4, by permission, July/August 1993. Copyright © 1993 by Health Forum, Inc.

The Power of Conscious, Active Learning

If you are a conscious, active learner in your approach to embracing the role shifts we've described in this book, you will take pains to understand yourself and your motivation. You become aware of what you want and need to learn. You invite feedback on your current leadership strengths and pinpoint opportunities for growth and development. You also engage in honest self-evaluation.

Ask yourself: *What do I know about myself right now? How will I seek further information and feedback?*

As an active learner, you develop learning *routines.* You might scan information sources regularly to keep up with changes in your field and in other fields that affect it. You might read the newspaper, browse professional journals, surf the Web to see what others are doing, take courses or workshops, listen to tapes while you drive or ride the train, and have lunch with a colleague from whom you can learn.

Ask yourself: *How much time do I spend learning?*

If you are an active learner, you open yourself to new ideas and techniques. You don't reject new approaches even if they feel uncomfortable and awkward. In fact, you consciously experiment with new ways of doing things.

Ask yourself: *When was the last time I created an experiment so I could learn from the experience?*

If you are an active learner, you make time or find time to learn, no matter how busy you are. You realize that every time people get together it is an opportunity to learn.

Ask yourself: *How do I take advantage of informal learning opportunities?*

If you're an active, avid learner, your colleagues, staff, friends, and family all know it, because it shows in the way you spend your time, the things you talk about, the questions you ask.

Ask yourself: *Do my friends view me as a role model of lifelong learning?*

If you're an active learner, you probably have a wish list of things you'd like to learn. Your desire to learn reveals itself in your thoughts. You think *I wish I had time to understand this or that better.* Or *I wish I could do this or that more quickly.* Or *I wish I could learn to do this myself without relying on someone else to do it.*

What if your organization's leaders were to say suddenly, "How about a two-month learning sabbatical?" Would you jump at the chance and hungrily entertain how many ways you might spend that precious time learning?

Ask yourself: *How hungry am I to learn?*

Take a Look at Yourself

As a brief exercise in self-reflection, let's give you a couple more questions to ask yourself (Exhibit 12.2).

Exhibit 12.2. Self-Reflection.

Self-reflection:

1. To what extent do I already demonstrate conscious active learning?
2. How do I demonstrate it?
3. How might *I* benefit by applying conscious active learning toward the roles identified in this book?

You Have an Opportunity

Since you've read this far, you probably feel some dissonance between your current ways of managing and the ten roles we've explored in this book. You may have identified roles that you want to strengthen, because you know that you have room to grow. That's a great beginning. The first giant step in becoming an even more active learner involves knowing what you want and need to learn. The next step involves figuring out how to get what you need. The final step involves believing in yourself and your ability to learn.

In this last chapter, we focus on three powerful ways you can consciously become a more active learner, and a more dynamic, successful, and ultimately indispensable leader (Exhibit 12.3).

Exhibit 12.3. Three Actions.

1. Focus your learning.
2. Decide how you learn best, and apply it.
3. Develop support for yourself and your learning.

Strategy One: Focus Your Learning

You've read about the ten role shifts and, we hope, bought (hook, line, and sinker) the point that strengthening them in yourself makes you not only more effective but also more gratified in your life.

How about taking a few minutes to crystallize precisely what it is you most want to strengthen (Exhibit 12.4)? As you read this book, which role shifts touch a chord in you, triggering the response that "the authors have got my number on this one; I need to do more of this"?

Exhibit 12.4. Ask Yourself.

Which shifts hold the most interest for you?

Which tools and techniques do you want to try?

In what ways do you think these ideas might help you and your team?

What thoughts have you had about yourself and your team as you read this book?

Which shifts, subjects, or skills do you want to learn more about?

Perhaps you already know what you want to apply and learn. However, if this doesn't feel clear to you, try the exercises in the remainder of this chapter to help you decide and commit.

⚒ Tool: A Tribute to You on Your Ninetieth

Purpose. This tool helps you identify your learning needs by seeing yourself as the kind of leader you want to become.

Method. Imagine it's your ninetieth birthday. People you've known over several decades are throwing you a party. The program for the evening engages people in sharing positive reflections about you *as a leader.*

On your ninetieth, what do you wish that each of the people listed in Exhibit 12.5 would say about your strengths and contributions as a leader during your lifetime? Would they say you are a go-getter, an inspiring coach, and a person who can really stimulate dialogue? What would you hope they say about you?

One more question. Between now and your ninetieth birthday, what skills, knowledge, qualities, or attitudes do you need to develop to *earn* these tributes about your strengths and contributions as a leader?

Exhibit 12.5. On Your Ninetieth.

	What You *Wish* They Would Say About Your Leadership
Your last boss	
Your closest family member or offspring	
One of your favorite work colleagues	
A close friend	
You yourself	

The answers give an important clue to the role shift(s) you want to achieve and the learning you'll most value as you continue growing into dynamic leadership.

Hard to figure out? How about asking people you respect to help you with this? Surveys abound that help managers learn how others (boss, staff, colleagues) perceive them. These 360 degree surveys can be helpful if you open yourself to the findings about you from the perspective of these various people. If your organization offers such a survey opportunity, seize the day and take advantage of it.

There are also a variety of leadership inventories and assessment tools that we have both used in our work. They generate invaluable information related to your leadership profile and are a wonderful way to get some objective data on your strengths and opportunity to grow.

In the meantime, try this straightforward interview with someone you trust and respect. We guarantee it will yield terrific information to help you further crystallize your leadership learning goals.

Tool: Interviews with Respected Others

Purpose. This tool solicits helpful feedback from people you trust, to further refine your learning plans.

Method. Look at the circle of people below. They have important—and differing—perspectives on you.

Your Circle of Influence

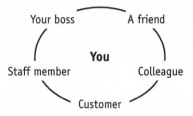

Select one person of each type, a person you respect who knows you well. Asking each person the questions below, you gain amazingly helpful perspective on your learning needs. Of course, you don't have to accept and act on what you hear; but listen, because you may decide you *want* to.

After these interviews, pore over your results and really think about them.

Interview Questions for Use with Respected Others

1. How would you describe my leadership or management style?
2. What are two things that you think I do particularly well?
3. What are two areas in which you think I could benefit from making changes or learning?
4. Please tell me about a situation in which you think I could have performed more effectively.

I'm going to show you a list of ten scales that describe alternative ways managers think and act. On each scale, I would like you to give me a rating to show where you think I fall.

1. Provider-oriented	1	2	3	4	5	Customer-focused
2. Silo thinking	1	2	3	4	5	Organizational thinking
3. Directing style	1	2	3	4	5	Coaching style
4. Status quo–oriented	1	2	3	4	5	Courageous, risk-taking, change-oriented

Interview Questions for Use with Respected Others (continued)

5. Oriented to keeping busy	1	2	3	4	5	Results-oriented
6. "Telling"	1	2	3	4	5	Facilitating dialogue
7. Protecting turf (or territorial)	1	2	3	4	5	Building relationships
8. Function manager	1	2	3	4	5	Business leader
9. Treats employees as expendable	1	2	3	4	5	Treats employees as precious
10. Appears pressured and overworked	1	2	3	4	5	Appears balanced, with perspective

If you were my learning coach, what would you suggest are areas I most need to develop?

Open yourself to what people told you about their perceptions of you. Imagine the consequences of following their advice about strengths you could benefit most from developing. Then focus your learning goals with the help of Exhibit 12.6.

Now that you've focused your learning, the next question is, How can you get what you need?

Exhibit 12.6. My Learning Target.

I recognize that active learning is the key to my future because

I am committing myself specifically to developing these strengths:

Most of all, I want to develop

Strategy Two: Decide How You Learn Best, and Apply It

Here we go again, advocating a *conscious* approach, this time to your learning process. It is our belief that if you consciously design your process, you can employ one that builds on your most positive experiences and strengths as a learner. You can plan a learning process that works for you, given your learning style and preferences.

To be concrete, here is a tool: our learning process preference audit. This audit lists a variety of the most popular (and we think most powerful) learning processes used by managers. In an effort to support your journey to personal mastery, consider each option and its appeal to you, given your learning targets. We're hoping this list helps you stretch your thinking, so that you consider the variety of learning methods available in selecting the one(s) most powerful and engaging for you.

✷ Tool: Learning Process Preference Audit

Purpose. This tool identifies optimal ways that you learn, so you can apply them as you continue to develop as a leader.

Method. Consider the list of learning process options in Exhibit 12.7. Think about how you learn best. Rate each one on its effectiveness for you, and the likelihood that it would energize you.

Next, draw conclusions. How might you pursue the optimal learning process for each of your goals? Tally your scores in each row.

Look at your scores, and identify those learning methods you find most powerful, given their effectiveness and your enthusiasm for them.

Now imagine how you can pursue the learning targets you identified earlier, using your favorite learning processes that you have just identified. This isn't quite as simple as it looks, because some learning processes are appropriate in pursuing some goals, but inappropriate for others. For instance, let's say your learning target is about becoming a more courageous change agent. You identified with the cases we outlined in Chapter Five, on courage, risk, and change, and you want to try some of the tools, but you have some concern based on past experiences. To help you learn and grow, reading, research, and investigation probably aren't going to work as well as getting a coach, or surrounding yourself with others who have success and experience to share.

Exhibit 12.7. Learning Process Options.

Learning Process Options	Effective for You? 1 = No, 5 = Yes	Energizing for You? 1 = No, 5 = Yes	Total Score
Coaching: Get a really good coach.			
Observation: Find positive examples and watch them closely. Do respectful and enthusiastic borrowing.			
Immersion: Surround yourself with people who are good at what you want to learn. Sit with them at lunch. Join them in discussion. Invite them to lunch.			
Feedback: Solicit honest feedback from others. Ask directed questions and probe for rich information about your performance. Ask for suggestions. Listen without being defensive.			
Postmortem: Analyze mistakes and disappointing results. They provide phenomenally rich learning opportunities. Open yourself to the dynamics that led to the result. Discuss alternatives.			
Retrospective review: After a meeting, project, or event, engage those involved in identifying what worked and what didn't and how to improve effectiveness for the future.			
Teach what you want to learn: Identify an employee who would benefit by what you yourself want to learn. Prepare to teach that employee the skill you want to build. Or become your staff's clipping service and circulate knowledge and skill-building goodies for all to see.			

Exhibit 12.7. (continued)

Learning Process Options	Effective for You? 1 = No, 5 = Yes	Energizing for You? 1 = No, 5 = Yes	Total Score
Hire a pro: Hire people with strengths you don't have. Appreciate and recognize those strengths, and learn from them.			
Project work: Volunteer to be second string on a related project.			
Cross lines: Organize or volunteer to serve on a task force that gives you cross-functional exposure.			
Step into the limelight: Take on a responsibility that makes you visible and puts pressure on you to figure out how to succeed.			
Do "far afield" trips: Arrange to visit people, programs, and services that are exemplary, and learn from them.			
Invite an observer: Ask a colleague to view your services and your performance with fresh eyes.			
Interview people: Ask people how they go about whatever it is you want to learn.			
Go public and ask for help: Tell people what you want to learn, and ask if they can help you.			
Try it: Experiment; learn from experience.			
Jump in: Step out of your comfort zone and into a responsibility or situation that forces you to stretch.			

Exhibit 12.7. (continued)

Learning Process Options	Effective for You? 1 = No, 5 = Yes	Energizing for You? 1 = No, 5 = Yes	Total Score
Read, research, and investigate: Surf the Web, hang out in bookstores, read books and journals, enter chatrooms, join listgroups, network with like-minded souls.			
Engage in formal learning: Go to school, take an online course, attend a workshop, let someone else do the planning.			

If your learning target is to become more focused on customers and skilled at satisfying them, your best bet might be taking some trips far afield, so to speak, that allow you to observe best practices in other respected organizations. Then, using this knowledge along with tools we've presented in this book, you can map out a plan, step up to the plate, and try it.

Using your audit results, consider how you *prefer* to learn. For each of your learning targets, consider which preferred learning approaches are appropriate to that target. So that you don't forget these amazing insights when you go grab for some potato chips, write them down using Exhibit 12.8.

By now, we hope you feel clarity about your stretch goals. In your quest to become an ever more effective leader, you know the role(s) you most want to learn, and you have decided on the learning process(es) that might serve you best in pursuit of your goals.

With an eye to easing your way, we recommend one further action. Once again, we suggest that you become conscious of who you are and what you need, as you proactively identify support for yourself in your learning process. Learning takes you out of your comfort zone and may trigger feelings of discomfort or anxiety. It helps immeasurably to have support that works for you.

Exhibit 12.8. Learning Targets and Means.

My Learning Target	How I Can Best Pursue It

Strategy Three: Develop Support for You and Your Learning

Let others in on your learning process. Learning doesn't have to be onerous, and you certainly don't have to tough it out alone. Permit others to coach you, remind you, check on you, or join you in your learning. Invite them to help you.

With people as busy as they are, you may need to take the initiative to amass support from others for your learning. The easiest way to accomplish this is simply to go public. Communicate your learning goals to your staff, your boss, and your colleagues. Tell them outright that you want their feedback and suggestions about your learning process and progress. Reassure them that you will welcome, not resent, their perceptions and ideas. Then thank them when they speak up (even if you don't like what they say).

Form a support group with other active learners. Use this group to solve problems, share ideas, or process experiences. Make sure you include managers with diverse skills and perspectives; that way, you can draw upon each other's strengths and abilities. This may be a stretch, and you and your group may experience discomfort and disagreements, but hang in there. We all learn a great deal from people who do not view the world exactly as we do.

Many of the organizations we have worked with formalize this concept and structure manager support groups for their entire leadership team. The groups become a safe place for leaders to process their learning and experience when they try on new leadership techniques and approaches. The main point is that learning is tough, and we need support when we hit the inevitable bumps in the road so that we don't give up.

But support from the outside isn't the only answer. Our last suggestion is to learn how to support yourself in your learning process. Most of us find it difficult to be completely objective. We tend to be either overly critical of our flaws and shortcomings or unaware of what we need to work on. We have already covered the concept of asking for help from others and discussed ways to use unbiased opinion to check our progress. The final, and probably the most important, support technique is to consciously watch, monitor, and celebrate your own journey.

We the authors both keep journals and try (although we know it is difficult) to process and critique important events. If we are designing a workshop, facilitating a retreat, or delivering a new speech, we make sure we put aside some quiet time to reflect on how we felt we did and what we could learn from the experience. We also know enough not to obsess on what we could have, or should have, done differently, but instead to balance critical analysis with positive acknowledgment. You will find your thinking shifting automatically and your ability to learn increasing tenfold when you feel good about yourself and your ability to learn and grow. So give yourself some positive affirmation.

Think about what you did right, what you are proud of, every day. These don't have to be large accomplishments, but it's easy to feel burnt out and overwhelmed if you only focus on what you didn't do. So brag, silently and out loud. Make sure you have people in your life who listen to you tell your success stories and who get pleasure out of watching you share these achievements.

Return the favor. Listen to their tales of glory. Form a group of positive-thinking survivors who know that although there are problems and challenges in being a learning and growing health care leader, optimism rather than pessimism is the healthy way to view one's role. Give yourself and those around you a boost and a break. After all, who wants to feel like wilted lettuce or a leaky boat when you can feel indispensable?!

References

Berwick, D. *Collaborative on Service Quality.* Boston: Institute for Healthcare Improvement, 1998.

"Implement the Balanced Scorecard and Become a Strategy-Focused Organization." Lincoln, Mass.: Balanced Scorecard Collaborative, 2001.

Kaplan, R., and Norton, D. *Balanced Scorecard: Translating Strategy into Action.* Cambridge, Mass.: Harvard Business School Press, 1996.

Kim, D. "The Leader with a Beginner's Mind." *Healthcare Forum Journal,* July-Aug. 1997, pp. 33–37.

Leebov, W., Scott, G., and Olson, L. *Achieving Impressive Customer Service.* Chicago: American Hospital Publishing, 1998.

Scott, G. "The Partnership Dialogue." Meadowbrook, Pa.: Gail Scott Associates, 1995.

Scott, G. "How Are You Feeling?" Meadowbrook, Pa.: Gail Scott Associates, 1996a.

Scott, G. "How Can We Mess This Up?" Meadowbrook, Pa.: Gail Scott Associates, 1996b.

Scott, G. "Monthly 'Bits.'" Meadowbrook, Pa.: Gail Scott Associates, 1996c.

Scott, G. "Success of the Week." Meadowbrook, Pa.: Gail Scott Associates, 1997a.

Scott, G. "Walk in the Shoes." Meadowbrook, Pa.: Gail Scott Associates, 1997b.

Scott, G. "What Will It Take?" Meadowbrook, Pa.: Gail Scott Associates, 1997c.

Scott, G. "Whom Do You Know?" Meadowbrook, Pa.: Gail Scott Associates, 1997d.

Scott, G. "How Do You Spend Your Time?" Meadowbrook, Pa.: Gail Scott Associates, 1999.

"The New Workforce: Generation Y." *Workplace Visions,* no. 2, 2001.

Workforce for the New Millennium. (HR Commission monograph.) Chicago: American Society for Healthcare Human Resources Administration, Nov. 2000.

Index

A

Achieving Impressive Customer Service (Leebov, Scott, and Olson), 23, 219
Act strategically strategy, 183, 186
Active learning, 245
Address your personal attitudinal blocks strategy, 230–234
Adjust your mind-set strategy, 153–157
Adjust your thinking strategy, 46–47
Adopt routine of scheduling priorities tool, 236–239
Advocacy tips, 220*e*
Advocate/remove obstacles strategy, 217–220
Aletha, 199
Alice, 199–200
Alternative intervention responses, 55*e*

B

Balanced perspective: benefits of, 229; as conscious choice, 242; instructive cases on, 226–227; issues/worries regarding, 227–228; need for, 225–226; questions for assessing focus on, 224–225; shift from pressure/overwork to, 9–10; strategies for achieving, 229–242
Balanced perspective strategies: address your personal attitudinal blocks, 230–234; be a living example of work-life balance, 240–242; learn to identify priorities, 234–235; listed, 230*e*
Balanced perspective toolkit, 230*e*
Balanced perspective tools: adopt routine of scheduling priorities, 236–239; be a work-life-balance role model, 241; be your own thought architect, 231–233; Fitting My Roles into My Schedule, 239*e*; "ligging," 233–234; My Most Important Roles, 238*e*; renovating your thoughts, 232*e*; role scheduling for work-life balance, 237–239*e*; self-reflection on work-life balance, 240–241; your urgency-importance matrix, 234–235
Be a living example of work-life balance strategy, 240–242
Be a work-life-balance role model, 241
Be your own thought architect tool, 231–233
Becoming skillful catalyst of dialogue strategy, 144–145*e*